TALES OF A COUNTRY OBSTETRICIAN

TALES OF A COUNTRY OBSTETRICIAN

UNFORGETTABLE STORIES ABOUT
PRACTICING MEDICINE IN ALABAMA

DANIEL M. AVERY, MD

iUniverse, Inc.
Bloomington

TALES OF A COUNTRY OBSTETRICIAN
Unforgettable Stories about Practicing Medicine in Alabama

iUniverse books may be ordered through booksellers or by contacting:

iUniverse
1663 Liberty Drive
Bloomington, IN 47403
www.iuniverse.com
1-800-Authors (1-800-288-4677)

ISBN: 978-1-4759-6322-9 (sc)
ISBN: 978-1-4759-6324-3 (hc)
ISBN: 978-1-4759-6323-6 (ebk)

Library of Congress Control Number: 2012922317

Printed in the United States of America

iUniverse rev. date: 12/05/2012

CONTENTS

This book is dedicated to the memory of John Roberts Faucette, PhD, MD, former chief of obstetrics at Carraway Methodist Medical Center in Birmingham, Alabama. Dr. Faucette was a master obstetrician/gynecologist and mentor to me during the time I was an OB-GYN resident. He treated his patients like they were his daughters, wife, or mother. He demanded only the best care for all, regardless of their socioeconomic status. He was the epitome of the caring physician and a model for the physician-patient relationship. As the profession goes, he was a "wizard with blades" and probably the best vaginal surgeon I have had the pleasure of working with. He treated the residents as sons and daughters, knowing each resident, spouse, and child by name. Dr. Faucette was the picture of great health, running five miles every day of his life, regardless of "sun, rain, sleet, or snow." He suffered a cardiac arrest and died while running outside St. Vincent's Hospital's emergency department in Birmingham, Alabama.

Dr. Faucette earned his PhD in neuroanatomy and taught in the anatomy department at the medical school for a number of years, after which he entered medical school. Being older, he was "picked on" by the residents and was often asked difficult questions in the operating room, as is often the case. During a complex vaginal reconstruction operation, the residents decided to call on John Faucette and ask him detailed questions about pelvic anatomy. The residents did not know he was a premier neuroanatomist. Dr. Faucette went through every fine detail of the anatomy of the pelvis. It was every medical student's dream. The attending physicians and residents were stunned. No one had any idea he was a seasoned neuroanatomist. It was great!

One Christmas season, I was scheduled to work both Christmas Eve and Day because one resident had lost both parents and another had a broken femur. Dr. Faucette came to me and reminded me I had two small children and a new baby and needed to be home on Christmas. I told him I would like to be but there was no one else to take my call (my on-duty shift). He told me he would take my call. I told him I couldn't let the division chief take call for a junior resident. He said it was an order and I had to obey him. He said if it made me feel any better, if he got busy, he would call me. Of course I never heard from him.

A gentleman, a scholar, a colleague, a mentor, and a friend, he will be missed. His memory will live on in those he cared for and those he trained. I am grateful for the opportunity to have trained with him.

PREFACE

Every physician who has ever practiced medicine has probably wished he or she had written down all the unusual, unbelievable, and hilarious things that happened to him or her throughout his or her career. Unfortunately, we usually don't. With time, these stories are usually lost. While we all experience these funny and unusual things, we usually regret not writing them. This book is a compilation of many of those stories. It has truly been enjoyable writing this book because it has allowed me to relive many experiences. It has been fun thinking about patients who have been in my life during the past thirty years. Without those patients, I not only wouldn't have any stories, I wouldn't have a career.

The things patients said often helped me get through the day after a long night of "call" or after a difficult situation with a patient or family. The thoughts behind many of these stories come from the patients themselves. Patients can be faithful, honorable, and true. Over the years, most of my patients have had my home phone number because getting in touch with me provided them security. Of the many who had my number, only a few abused the privilege. Often, a simple "thank you" from a patient made my entire day worthwhile.

Writing this book has allowed me to enjoy my patients for the rest of my life, even after I retire. Those written memories can never be taken from me. Even if my memory fails, I can still read my book and enjoy it.

I appreciate the encouragement of my longtime partner, Dr. Dwight E. Hooper, who encouraged me to write these stories and publish this book.

INTRODUCTION

I was born in 1950 at DCH Regional Medical Center in Tuscaloosa, Alabama, where I grew up. I spent a lot of time in the doctor's office as a child because I was sickly. Our pediatrician once thought I had polio, but I eventually got well from whatever was wrong with me. One of my high school coaches recently told me he was floored I had become a doctor. No one thought I would ever make anything of myself.

I wanted to be a doctor as long as I can remember. There had never been a doctor in my family. Most of my family had been in the railroad business. I did not know how much money physicians made, but I knew they made sick patients well. My father died when I was a teenager, and I thought this would close the door on any opportunities for becoming a physician.

I have had many life experiences that made me interested in becoming a physician. I was intrigued by ambulances, and during my teens, I worked for a funeral home chain that owned an ambulance service. I saw a lot of sick and injured patients and got to spend time in the emergency departments of hospitals. The funeral home served as the morgue for the medical examiner's autopsies. I learned a lot about anatomy there. After college, I went to physician assistant school and worked for a hospital and then the Department of Forensic Sciences.

The real opportunity to learn medicine came with medical school. However, getting in the door was a formidable task. I applied three times before getting accepted. The dean of admissions told me I would never get into the University of Alabama School of Medicine. He said it cost twenty-five dollars to apply and that I should not waste my money. He suggested I do something useful with my money—like taking my wife out to eat.

But I got in, and medical school turned out to be a lot of work. I had to work part-time on the side. My wife had two jobs. I was excited to be in medical school, but it was far more work than I had ever dreamed!

Residency was even more work. Instead of paying tuition, interns actually got paid a salary. It was hectic, stressful, exhausting, sometimes humiliating, occasionally embarrassing, and oftentimes demanding. "Attendings" (an attending physician is one who has completed residency and practices medicine in a clinic or hospital in the specialty learned during residency) wanted you to go home and read, but sometimes it was all you could do to hold your head up. Overall, it was a great but strenuous experience.

One of my best educational experiences during residency was working at Pickens County Medical Center in Carrollton, Alabama. I learned a lot and got to do a lot. Most of what I learned, I learned on the spot because it was immediately necessary, and no one else was around to help me. Many things I did for the first time without assistance while reading from a book or talking to someone on the telephone.

Private practice was an eye-opening experience, especially for a chief resident who thought he knew everything. Fortunately, I continued to learn. Most of all, I learned I did not know everything. It has been as much work as residency.

My greatest contribution to medicine has been practicing in rural Alabama. I started practicing medicine in the Carraway Northwest Medical Center emergency department in Winfield, Alabama, during residency, working part-time in obstetrics and gynecology after residency until moving there permanently after fellowship training. The hospital was new and had state-of-the-art labor and delivery suites, central monitoring and equipment, and anesthesia services in the hospital all the time. I would never have left there had the hospital not stopped obstetric services and the malpractice insurance carrier gone bankrupt.

The final chapter in my life appears to be practicing medicine at the University of Alabama School of Medicine in Tuscaloosa, Alabama. What an honor! I applied to be a faculty member four times over my career before being accepted. I have had the pleasure of serving as the chair of obstetrics and gynecology, the chief of staff, and the president of the joint medical staffs at DCH Regional Medical Center. I have been able to maintain my rural practice. I have been practicing part-time or full-time in Winfield, Alabama, since 1982. It has been an honor to train those students and residents who will provide medical care after I am gone.

As I look back, my career has been rewarding and worthwhile. Every day, medical students ask me, "If you had it to do again, would you still be a physician?" Without any hesitation, I answer, "Yes!"

I

I'VE WANTED TO BE A DOCTOR
SINCE I WAS A YOUNG BOY

Ever since I was a young boy, I've wanted to be a doctor. During medical school, my mother gave me a picture of me dressed up as a doctor. My dad had brought me a play doctor's kit from a business trip, and I used one of my mother's white blouses to make a lab coat. I had an ENT light strapped to my head, a stethoscope around my neck, and I carried a doctor's bag. I was ready to practice.

Padded Bras and the Middle School Rose Ball

All girls in elementary school have "cooties"—whatever that is. It's interesting, though, that in middle school those same girls begin to look pretty good. Curves and breasts seem to come out of nowhere, and you wonder how you could have missed them a year earlier. Not every girl develops at the same time. Every girl in class had a bra, but not every girl had something to put into it. This is where padded bras came in. Even girls with nothing could look like Marilyn Monroe in three quick snaps.

The Rose Ball was the middle school version of the high school prom. Students got dressed up and danced with one another. It was only square dancing, but it was still fun. A female classmate and I were dancing. I could not remember from school who had breasts and who did not. This girl did not, but I did not know that. After a few quick turns, I bumped her left breast and accidentally turned the padded cup inside out. It looked really strange. She didn't notice, but I sure did! I didn't know what to do. Should I squeeze the cup and try to pop it out, or should I leave it alone? Several girls in my class saw what had happened and took the girl to the restroom so they could fix her bra. I was rescued!

Stimulating Bowel Function

I dated Sandra during middle school and high school. Each summer, the youth choir went on a tour, usually traveling to some far-off area of the United States. This trip involved spending a fair amount of time on a bus. Sandra and I usually sat together on the trips, since we were "going together." (I was never sure where we were going.) Sandra loved Chiclets gum. During a stop to let everyone use the restroom and get something to drink, I decided to buy some gum and made an interesting discovery. Chiclets look exactly like Feen-a-Mint laxatives. They are also about the same size. So I bought both and swapped the gum pieces.

When we got back on the bus, I laid my pack of "Chiclets" on the seat. Sandra picked them up and ate one . . . two . . . three . . . four pieces!

The directions on the box said, "Bowel stimulation begins in about an hour." Suddenly there was a mad rush to the bus restroom. Sandra got diarrhea on the bus, and I felt really bad. But the worst thing I did was tell her what I had done, because then she had diarrhea and was angry.

Tanner Staging of the Breasts

I grew up with a beautiful girl named Rose. She remains a lifelong friend. Now we are both sixty, and she is still a very attractive woman. She was always bright and friendly. She was a cheerleader at our high school and was active in everything, including our church.

Our youth group from church went camping at Camp Tuscoba one weekend. The girls slept on one side of the hill and the boys on the other. Each shared a set of bathrooms. One group sat by the campfire while the other showered. Then we alternated. Of course the girls got to go first.

One night, as the boys sat by the campfire and the girls showered, one of the girls left the bathroom door wide open in clear view of the boys about twenty feet away. Rose had just gotten out of the shower and was drying off. There she was, without a stitch on. I did not know girls looked like that and I was never the same . . . I knew I would be a gynecologist one day.

Shark Attack or Menstrual Bleeding?

I had no sisters, only a brother, and I knew nothing about menses, or "periods." We grew up in a prim and proper, strict Baptist home. Sex, girls, and contraception were not mentioned.

In the tenth grade, I went with my girlfriend's church youth group to Gulf Shores, Alabama. Most everybody I knew from school, and there were only a few chaperones. I thought this would be a fun time, and the first two days were filled with good meals in the dining hall and a lot of kissing on the beach before bedtime. The boys slept in one building and the girls in another.

But disaster struck on day three. We all went to the beach to swim and "catch some rays." A girl my age, who was pleasant and smart, was swimming in the Gulf of Mexico. She had on a white one-piece bathing suit. When she came out of the water, blood and clots were pouring out of her bathing suit and down her leg. All of us guys had the same immediate thought: she had been bitten by a shark and was bleeding profusely. We started running toward her but were stopped by the girls. They told us we could not go near her, but we told them that she had been bitten by a shark and needed to go to the hospital.

My girlfriend said, "No!" The girls were going to take her to her room and would take care of her. I knew they did not know how to sew skin and was sure they had no medical equipment with them, like sutures. We guys were stunned. The girls surrounded her, and they disappeared to her room. We did not see her again until we went home. That night, instead of kissing on the beach after dinner, my girlfriend introduced me to the world of menstrual periods. It was nauseating and made me dizzy.

What really got me, though, was when she said this happened every month! I said, "You have got to be kidding!" Guys certainly do not do this. I did not recall blood and clots pouring out of me every month, and I think I would have noticed that. I was still skeptical. When I got home from the trip I asked my mom about this. My brother did not have periods that I knew of. My mother laid it out for me. It was true. So I asked my grandmother, and she said it had to do with sin and eating of the fruit of life in the book of Genesis in the Bible. I was even more confused.

Dancing Leads to Intercourse

Growing up in a strict Baptist home, there was no dancing of any kind allowed, not even square dancing. When I was in the fifth grade, I was so embarrassed because I was the only kid who could not dance. So I questioned my mother about why I could not dance at school.

She said, "Dancing leads to other things."

I asked, "Like what?"

She said she could not tell me.

I asked, "How would I know if dancing was leading to other things?"

She replied, "Just don't dance."

Eventually, as we got older, she let us square dance in school.

Some forty-five years later, I thought about the dancing at school and asked my mother about it. I asked if she was implying that dancing could lead to sex, and she said yes. I asked her what she thought the odds were of dancing leading to sex in the elementary school classroom, where we could only square dance with the teacher standing right by us.

She said, "You never know."

I am reminded of the old story that Baptists do not have sex standing up because someone might think they were dancing!

Last week, our church announced it would start having dancing lessons on Wednesday nights.

Hypothermia at the First Baptist Church

Baptists and a few other faiths practice complete immersion of converts in what is called a baptistery. Baptisteries are pools deep enough to stand in and are visible to the congregation. Those being baptized wear thin white cotton gowns furnished by the church, along with their own underwear. In the summer, the water is room temperature. But in the winter, the water is cold unless hot water is added. As soon as the morning worship service was over, the water was turned on because it took all afternoon to fill the baptistery for the evening baptisms. My teenage buddies and I had a friend who was going to be baptized at the evening service. It was late January.

My buddies had an idea. After the morning service was over and everyone had gone, my buddies slipped into the baptistery area and turned off the hot water, leaving only cold water flowing. By the end of the afternoon, the baptistery pool was full. The minister wore a gown that was lined with a rubber suit. He did not realize the water was so cold, but our friend did!

"Cardioversion" for Not Knowing Bible Verse

I dated Sandra through middle school and some of high school. After that, she started dating a very large guy from another class who did not like me, probably because I had dated Sandra.

At Baptist Training Union, three people were asked Bible verses. We sat in front of the group on stools. I did not know the stools had been wired to a metal plate on the seat that was attached to a power cord. Those who did not answer the questions correctly would get shocked. My turn came, and I was asked when motorcycles were mentioned in the Bible.

I had no idea, and the moderator, who happened to be the big guy, replied, "And Joshua rode on to Jericho." I thought the verse didn't say anything about a motorcycle.

Then it happened: I received 120 volts through my buttocks, knocking me off the stool and onto the floor.

It just did not seem the appropriate thing to do in church.

II

WORKING AS A FUNERAL DIRECTOR AND EMERGENCY MEDICAL TECHNICIAN

My first introduction to medicine was employment by a funeral home chain that owned an ambulance service. Before 1970, ambulance companies were typically owned by funeral homes and shared employees. There was no standardized training of ambulance attendants until 1970. Embalming provided an opportunity to learn anatomy, disease processes, and visualize trauma. The funeral home where I worked had a large embalming area and morgue where the medical examiner often performed autopsies. This was where I learned anatomy before medical school. I found this experience intriguing, and it stimulated my desire to become a doctor.

Wheels Fall off Ambulance on Emergency Run

In the late 1960s, a national interest began with the emergency care and transportation of the sick and injured, culminating in a federal act in 1970, creating emergency medical technicians (EMTs). There were grants for training and certifying EMTs and for producing equipped ambulances. The first ambulances produced were 1969 High Top Pontiac ambulances. There were equipped to carry four patients and they had a Federal coaster siren and many flashing red lights. Unfortunately, the electrical system was not powerful enough to supply lights and a siren at night when the headlights and taillights were on, so to run the siren, the headlights would go almost dim.

However, the biggest problem with these ambulances was that the chassis was not strong enough to support the modifications. The end result was that at higher speeds, the back wheels often fell off. One day, while running an emergency in town, I noticed the driver's side back wheel was situated way out from the wheel well. Shortly after, that wheel completely separated from the ambulance and rolled down the middle of the street right past me. Of course the back of the chassis crashed to the ground, and we slowed to a stop. We called for another ambulance. My attendant in the back replied, "This happens all the time."

Stretcher Falls out of Ambulance

Ambulance stretchers are held securely in the back of an ambulance, hearse, first call vehicle, or rescue unit by what are called "cot hooks." These devices lock the stretcher firmly in place. If not secured, the stretcher will roll around, and with the weight of a patient, they can be hard to manage. The stretcher could also topple and injure the patient. Depending on the manufacturer, stretchers weigh between fifty and seventy pounds.

One time, after delivering a patient to the hospital and in a hurry to get back to business, the attendants quickly put an empty stretcher into the back of the ambulance. Unfortunately, they did not properly close the back door. When they drove off, the stretcher came unlatched and rolled around in the back of the ambulance. The stretcher hit the back door, and the weight of it knocked the door open. The stretcher fell onto the pavement. Fortunately, no one was injured.

Blowing the Engine in an Ambulance

Before 1971, most funeral homes had ambulance services and they shared employees. Funeral homes had an ambulance service because if a patient died on an ambulance run, a funeral home had an interest in trying to handle the business. In 1969, an ambulance trip in town cost $17.50, with an additional $2.50 if it was an emergency. A funeral cost as much as $3,000 to $4,000. Money was not in the ambulance business.

The funeral home where I worked had four ambulances: two high-top Pontiacs and two converted station wagons (a Pontiac and a Buick). The station wagons were generally used for house calls for one patient and the high tops for automobile accidents because they could carry four patients on stretchers: two lying down and two "hanging" from ceiling supports. Ambulances age very quickly because of excessive mileage and fast, hard driving. Most accumulate two hundred thousand miles while in service for only a few years.

Another attendant and I made a house call for a patient who the family said appeared dead. We took the call in the oldest ambulance we had because it was the only one available. It was a worn-out 1969 Pontiac high top. We ran an emergency, and the trip there went well. After loading the patient, we ran to the hospital. Just inside the city limits, the engine started making an awful sound and smoke poured out of the double exhausts. The engine slowed. I radioed the ambulance company base, but the dispatcher said all other vehicles were on runs and to try to make it to the hospital, which was approximately two miles away. We were moving so slowly I cut off the lights and siren because everyone was passing us.

We were half a block from the hospital when the engine died. The hospital was straight ahead in clear view, so we decided to take the stretcher out of the ambulance and run along University Boulevard to the emergency department. We told the man's wife to walk to the emergency room, and away we went. I was in front and Robert, the other attendant, was in the back. I think people got out of our way just out of curiosity. We made it to the hospital.

Then I called the owner of the ambulance company and funeral home and said, "Mr. Hayes, this is Danny. I blew up number 10!"

What Is in the Back of a Hearse?

People are always curious about hearses and what is in the back of them, knowing good and well that it is usually a deceased body. If there is a stretcher in the back of a hearse and it is covered with a sheet, blanket, or cot cover, chances are it is a deceased person. Nevertheless, everyone always wants to look through the windows in the back and see what is there.

When I worked for the funeral home, some of the most curious people were gasoline attendants, now mostly a thing of the past. As they pumped gasoline, they would get a close-up view of what was in the back of the hearse. They always asked who was in the back, how the person had died, and worse, if they could see the body. It was annoying and really inappropriate.

One evening, after making a trip to another city, we needed gasoline. We pulled off the road, and one of my colleagues got onto the stretcher, and I covered him with a blanket, leaving only a hand exposed. We then drove to the service station.

While pumping gas, the attendant told me he thought he saw the hand of the body move. I told him that was impossible because the person was dead. He kept on, so one of the guys opened the back of the hearse. The ambulance attendant under the cover sat up and grabbed the gas attendant, scaring him nearly to death. The gas attendant never again asked questions about what was in the back of the hearse.

Patient Steals Ambulance at Mental Hospital

I can still hear the dispatcher clearly telling us, "When you go to a mental hospital to pick up a patient, always turn the engine off, take out the keys, and lock the vehicle. Patients will steal the ambulance." Of course we never thought it would happen to us, but it did. It was disheartening after loading the patient onto the stretcher inside the hospital and rolling him outside, only to discover the ambulance was gone. So we called the dispatcher and told him what had happened. Worse still, we had to call the police and report a stolen ambulance.

Fortunately, the ambulance was later found undamaged. We locked the vehicles and took the keys with us after that.

Ambulance Runs to Sorority Houses

Paramedics and EMTs have an understood priority of ambulance runs. The lowest priority call is transportation of a deceased body, which is never an emergency because the opportunity to render care has passed. The next priority calls are nursing home and residential transfers, which could become an emergency if the patient is sicker than previously thought. The next priority run is the class of emergencies. Most paramedics and EMTs prefer emergency runs because that means red lights, sirens, and speed. A house call for an emergency is acceptable but not nearly the same as a multiple car accident, which may involve several ambulances.

The highest priority ambulance run is a call to a sorority house at the local university. Paramedics and EMTs fistfight, pull rank, or play like it is a transfer and leave the station with red lights and siren on. Often, two crews in one ambulance or in two ambulances might show up at a sorority house. Why are these so popular? Think about it. Calls are usually at night when the sorority girls are there. The calls are usually for syncope (fainting), falls, or seizures. And most of the girls are in nightgowns and pajamas—or less.

Ambulance Attendant Left at the Scene

Ambulance Service Company was called by the Tuscaloosa Police Department to respond to a motor vehicle accident on Tenth Avenue at Seventeenth Street. There was one injury. A driver and attendant responded in a smaller ambulance that could carry two patients if need be. The ambulance was a modified Pontiac station wagon.

The team arrived and secured the patient on the stretcher and loaded it into the back of the ambulance. In a hurry, the driver ran around to the driver's side, got in, and sped off, leaving the attendant standing at the back of the ambulance. I am sure those watching nearby did not understand what was happening, but the police caught on quickly. The driver did not notice that he was by himself until arriving at the hospital emergency department. The attendant back at the scene slipped into the crowd and walked back to the ambulance company.

Patient Falls out of Ambulance

Most ambulance stretchers require two people to operate. There are also "one-man stretchers" that can be operated, loaded, and unloaded by a single person. When the front wheels of the one-man stretcher are rolled into the vehicle, the legs collapse and the stretcher rolls right in. The reverse is considerably more complicated because if the front legs do not catch when the stretcher is pulled out of the ambulance, the front end of the stretcher falls to the ground, dumping the patient onto the surface below.

We had a transfer from one hospital to another hospital, and we had to use a one-man stretcher. Everything went well until we got to our destination and unloaded. The front legs did not catch, and the front end of the stretcher fell to the pavement. Fortunately, the patient stayed on the stretcher mattress, which slid up under the ambulance. Thank goodness the engine was off.

The ambulance entrance to the hospital was on one of the busiest streets in the town. A lot of people passing by got to see ambulance attendants on their stomachs, trying to "snake" the patient out from under the ambulance. Most of them just laughed at us. The patient was unharmed.

Picking Up a Patient and Finding a Surprise Underneath

Picking up patients from hospital beds and putting them on stretchers requires training. Two ambulance attendants have to distribute themselves alongside the patient, roll the patient toward themselves, and then lift the patient onto the stretcher. One has to be careful about blindly sliding his hand up under a patient because a surprise often resides there. Sure enough, we were in a hurry to move a patient and did not look beneath the patient as we were instructed. I felt the "surprise," and there was no question about what it was. My hand smelled awful all day despite washing it many times.

Ambulance Attendant Tries to Kiss Patient

Ambulance Service Company was called to a house in the county where a man was having chest pain. We made the call in a high-top Pontiac ambulance that was partially equipped. There was one trained EMT on board and another in training. The more experienced attendant drove and the less experienced man took care of the patient, which is the opposite of protocol today. We made an emergency run to the house, loaded the patient, and headed to the hospital, with clearance from the police and sheriff's offices as an emergency. In other words, we had police permission to exceed the speed limit with red lights and siren.

We were moving about ten miles per hour faster than traffic, with red lights and siren on. As we neared the city limits, John, my attendant, slid back the glass between us and said, "Hit it! He's arrested and I am starting CPR!" There was no bag mask apparatus, and CPR had to be done mouth to mouth. John did not know that the patient had simply fallen asleep. All of a sudden I heard yelling and saw my attendant and the patient fistfighting in the back. I pulled off the road, stopped the ambulance, and opened the back door.

I asked, "What are y'all doing?"

The patient replied, "Your attendant was trying to kiss me!"

Patient Too Big to Ride in an Ambulance

Ever think about what happens when a patient is too large to ride in an ambulance? Most ambulance stretchers will hold someone weighing up to 325 pounds. As America gets fatter, many people exceed that amount. Today, there are newer, heavier-duty stretchers, but patients weighing more than 500 pounds are still a challenge. When people get up to 1,000 pounds or more, they are unable to fit inside an ambulance. A recent patient who weighed about 1,100 pounds needed to go to the hospital for acute care. He could not fit through the door of his house, and a wall had to be removed to get him out. Flatbed trucks, wrecker trucks, and pickup trucks are often necessary to transport these people.

So what do you put these people on? How do you carry them? The answer is, the best that you can, with whatever you can.

Ambulance Driver Stops at Restaurant to Eat

Emergency runs are by far the most popular because of speed, red lights, the siren, and excitement. I was asked to go as an attendant with a senior attendant/driver on an out-of-town transfer from a nursing home forty-five miles away. On those calls, attendants just try to make the best of it.

After we got beyond the city limits, the driver "hit it," or started driving fast. Bear in mind we were running without red lights and siren. I asked why we were going so fast.

He said, "This is the plan. We'll get there as soon as we can. We're going to stop for supper at a restaurant just before we get to where have been dispatched. We'll eat chicken because it can be fixed quickly."

I said I was not sure about all this. The senior attendant replied it would not take any more time and the call was not an emergency.

We got to the restaurant, parked the ambulance in the woods, and went in and ate. Then we hurried and picked up the patient. The nursing home staff said they had called the ambulance company back and asked what was taking so long. The senior attendant said the traffic was heavy and we were not running an emergency. Unfortunately, the patient was the grandfather of one of my friends, and I felt bad.

Ambulance Runs in a Hearse

There were hearses long before there were ambulances. The sick have been transported by all methods of travel. They were carried on pallets in the Bible. In the old West, the sick and injured were often carried on horseback or in the back of a horse-drawn wagon. As a little girl, my grandmother had a serious eye injury and was carried by train from rural Alabama to a hospital in Montgomery. During the last century, it was apparent that most hearses were station wagon–like vehicles and could carry a stretcher, making them usable to carry the sick and injured. Even after the invention of ambulances, there were still emergency vehicles known as "combinations," which were combinations of hearses and ambulances.

Before 1970, it was not uncommon to see a hearse or "combination" making an emergency ambulance call. A siren was mounted under the hood, and occasionally there would be a rotating red light that could be placed on the roof; otherwise, emergencies had to be run with headlights on bright to warn other motorists. People did not think twice about seeing a hearse responding to an emergency. We commonly ran ambulance calls in hearses, especially nonemergency calls or transfers. If a hearse was parked outside a residence, it was apparent someone has passed away or was sick and needed to go to the hospital. Today, people would probably be terrified to ride to the hospital in a hearse. Times change . . .

"I Need an Ambulance, but Don't Bring That %$@*! Red Truck"

In 1970, the Federal Emergency Care and Transportation of the Sick and Injured Act changed emergency care in the field forever. Ambulance attendants and drivers had to be trained and certified. Ambulances had to meet specifications and be appropriately equipped.

Our ambulance company bought the first well-equipped ambulance available at the time. It was a raised-roof Chevrolet Suburban with a 450 HP high-performance engine—in other words, it would "fly." It had all kinds of equipment for patient care and would accommodate a regular stretcher and three portable stretchers. You could "lay two and hang two." One portable stretcher could lie beside the regular stretcher, and the other two hung from hooks from the ceiling. Two were "downstairs" and two were "upstairs," so to speak. The Chevrolet Suburban had a new electronic siren and several red lights. Nearly everyone in health care thought this was a great advance; unfortunately, society did not see it that way.

People did not like electronic sirens because they didn't "sound right." They believed the truck ambulance was a disgrace to the profession; a limousine-style Cadillac or Pontiac was more appropriate. People did not like medical care on the scene; they were more accustomed to the "scoop and run" technique. People would call for an ambulance and say, "I need an ambulance, but don't bring that %$@*! red truck!"

The Two Fears of Funeral Directors

Over centuries, funeral directors have had two great fears: misidentification of a body and embalming someone who is still alive. Nothing is worse than opening the casket for the first time only to hear the family say, "That is not our grandmother!" Sometimes just the process of embalming with restorative art actually improves the appearance of a body. When bodies are picked up from the hospital, they may be insufficiently identified. Sometimes the funeral home may pick up a body at a hospital or nursing home and return to the funeral home, failing to tag the body. Suits have occurred over misidentification of a body.

Far worse and rarely divulged by the profession is embalming someone who is still alive. Embalmers rarely discuss this issue. Before 1970, anyone in Alabama could pronounce someone dead. One could go into Grandmother's room, and if there was no movement or palpable pulse, just call the funeral home and tell them Grandmother had passed away. They would come pick her up, take her to the funeral home, and embalm her. Before 1950, the attendant would actually come to one's house and embalm the body there in the bed. They returned the following day and positioned the body in a casket.

Often one thinks a body is dead when it is actually in a coma, hypotensive (has abnormally low blood pressure), or such. A "cut down" is done to pump embalming fluid throughout the vascular system. The embalming fluid is a stimulant, and it is apparent for a short period of time that the body is alive until the formalin kills the tissue. One thing is always true—if embalming fluid is injected, the body will be dead soon if not already. Sometimes, at the cut down, bleeding from vessels may indicate the body is still alive.

Today, the pendulum has swung to the other extreme. In 1970, anyone could pronounce someone dead. Now, only a few can pronounce someone dead at home. If you call and report the death of Grandmother at home, no one will accept anyone's diagnosis, even that of a physician. Instead, an ambulance, fire engine, rescue vehicle, battalion chief, and police show up with red lights burning and sirens blaring, only to say, "Grandmother is dead." Worse yet, if not under hospice care, a homicide investigation is initiated. It is unfortunate that a new EMT's opinion supersedes that of a physician.

Patient Thrown into the Snow and Pronounced Dead

When there is motor vehicle accident (MVA), ambulances may be summoned by bystanders, the police, or the fire department. One freezing, snowy evening, our ambulance company received a call from the local police for assistance at an MVA in downtown Tuscaloosa. The dispatcher said there were eight injuries and one fatality. Any information would allow the ambulance service to know how much equipment to send on any particular call. With eight injuries, three ambulances were dispatched, each with two attendants. Two high-top ambulances would carry four patients apiece and a smaller ambulance two patients. All three vehicles were running emergencies authorized by the police with red lights and siren. A funeral home attendant alone was dispatched to the scene in a hearse to pick up the deceased patient.

The fatality had been thrown from her automobile and had been lying in the snow for some time. Once pronounced dead, attention was directed to those still alive. In 1968, anyone could pronounce a patient dead in Alabama because there were no rules regarding this. No movement, pulse, or evidence of life could be detected. So the fatality was loaded onto a stretcher and transported to the funeral home. The fatality was placed on the embalming table. The rest of the night crew was carrying injured patients to the hospital. When everyone was back from the call, the patient would be embalmed.

Several hours passed before the funeral director returned to the preparation room. The room was fairly warm. When it got time to inject the body with embalming solution, the embalmer noticed that his incision for embalming caused bleeding. He soon realized she was still alive but perhaps in a coma and unresponsive. She was quickly loaded onto an ambulance stretcher and received as best resuscitative care as possible in a funeral home. She was taken by ambulance to the hospital running an emergency with red lights and siren. She died at the hospital two weeks later from head injuries sustained in the MVA. She was probably one of only a few persons ever resuscitated by an embalmer.

Big Safety Pins on Ambulance Calls

As a new ambulance attendant, I was mentored by Jim, a law student who was also a student at the University of Alabama. We did the very first EMT course together and usually worked together. Working for the ambulance company was a great job because I could go to school during the day and study at night when we were not busy. Jim carried a large safety pin attached to his shirt; it was always there. I asked him what it was for, and he told me he would show me sometime.

Some of the most difficult calls were those to the old mansions in downtown Tuscaloosa, where the old homes were three or four stories high. Most of the homes had stairs with multiple flights. One Sunday night, we got the inevitable call to an old home on University Boulevard. A middle-aged woman on the third floor was sick and needed to go to the hospital. We went into the residence with the stretcher and looked up the long stairway. We went up the stairs and found a very large lady who was not very cooperative. I asked Jim if we were going to have to carry this three-hundred-pound woman down all those stairs. The stretcher alone weighed seventy pounds.

Jim said he would show me what his safety pin was for. He told me to get on one side of the woman and he got on the other. He stuck her with the pin, she jumped up, and we grabbed her and walked her down the stairs to the stretcher.

Homemade Ambulance

Working as an EMT was one of the most rewarding experiences I have ever had. If the pay had been better, I would never have gone to medical school. Over the years, I have reminisced about the exciting, often lifesaving calls that provided me a small living. As the years passed, I had a great idea: build a super-equipped ambulance and staff it with the physicians and nurses in the neighborhood. It would be a neighborhood service.

The ambulance design was based on a low-top Ford Explorer, which already had split seats in the back. I bought a Ferno Washington portable stretcher, which would fit in the back compartment of the Explorer with adequate headroom. It had retractable wheels and could roll in and out of the SUV. The engine was a V8 with plenty of power. I installed a multifunction electronic siren under the hood so it would be disguised. The control box was mounted inside the cab. When it came time to get red lights, I went to the emergency equipment supply store in downtown Birmingham. The store had red flashing lights but also green, clear, orange, and even black. I asked what the black lights were for but no one knew.

So I did what I thought was right: I bought some of all the colors. I wired the siren and multiple lights into the electrical system of the Explorer. Somewhere along the way, I got the wires crossed in the electrical harness. The siren would only work if I had the radio in the dash on. The red lights would only work if the windshield wipers were on and running. I then installed a cell phone in the front by the driver and one in the back by the attendant. The vehicle also had a CB radio in the front. At this point, the truck looked peculiar, but I continued to equip it. In the stretcher area, I had every possible piece of equipment to render care. I ordered a nitrous oxide cylinder, but it never came.

What would really make my ambulance legitimate would be to have it certified by the state EMS board. So I called the board and explained to them what I had done and my ideas for a neighborhood ambulance service. After telling the inspector my whole story, there was a long pause on the other end of the phone.

Then I heard him say, "You did what? We cannot certify that!"

So I hung up.

III

WORKING IN FORENSIC PATHOLOGY

After college, I worked as a physician assistant in pathology for the Department of Forensic Sciences. During medical school, pathology residency, and some of my career, I worked for the medical examiner's office.

"I Don't Want You to Get Hurt in the Autopsy Room"

The chief of pathology at the hospital was trained during an earlier generation, in which an autopsy was performed with a keenly sharpened fifteen-inch butcher knife. At the end of his autopsies, blood was everywhere—on the walls, the ceiling, the floor, and on the assistants. The pathologist would wave his knife as he cut tissue. I remember that famous line, in which he warned his medical students: "Stand back—I don't want you to get hurt!"

William Gives Preoperative Urine and Blood Samples

My brother-in-law was scheduled to have a tonsillectomy at the hospital where I worked as a physician assistant. He was told that he needed preoperative labs the day before surgery and to come the hospital after school. Knowing he would need to give a urine specimen, his mother told him not to urinate all day, which he did with difficulty. So when he arrived, he needed to urinate very badly. The lab technician let him give the urine specimen first. He was told to go into the restroom and fill the cup with urine. He filled one cup, then another, and then another until he had filled seventeen cups full of urine. He left the restroom, and the technician told him to bring the cup to the work counter. William told the tech he would need some help bringing the urine because he had filled seventeen cups. The tech said he only needed one. William said he had not been told how many cups to fill.

Then it was time for blood to be drawn. William had never had blood drawn before. The technician collecting was new. He stuck William with a Vacutainer in the brachial artery, allowing blood to spew about two feet into the air. The technician put his hand on the stream and worked it down to the needle and put on a tube to catch the blood. Both the technician and William had blood all over them.

William later asked me, "Is that the way they usually draw blood?"

Dinner with a Famous Forensic Pathologist

Herman Douglas Jones, PhD, was the first forensic pathologist in Alabama. He founded the Alabama Department of Toxicology and Criminal Investigation in 1926. Later he moved to Atlanta, Georgia, to found the medical examiner's office. He remained in Atlanta until his retirement in the mid-1970s. In 1975 he moved back to Alabama, where he served as consulting forensic pathologist for the Department of Forensic Sciences until his death in the late-1970s. A gentleman and scholar, Dr. Jones was magnificent even in the sunset of his career. He was known internationally, and a number of books have been written about him.

We became close friends working together, and we often had dinner together. One day, I arrived at the Jones's home for dinner, and Mrs. Jones announced that we were having Dr. Jones's favorite delicacy. I thought, *What could it be? Filet mignon, steak Oscar, chicken divan?*

Mrs. Jones delivered two plates to the table with pickled pig's feet on both. I was speechless. Then I felt nauseated. I sat for a while without saying anything, and Dr. Jones caught on very quickly.

He said, "You don't like pig's feet, do you?"

I said, "Dr. Jones, I don't. Could I make a peanut butter sandwich?"

District Attorney Falls Asleep in Court

While working for the Alabama Department of Forensic Sciences, a significant part of my job was providing testimony in court. While listening to others testify was very interesting, my own experience on the stand was not pleasant. The work of defense attorneys is to destroy witnesses' credentials and discredit their testimony, if what they say hurts the defense of their client. I can remember going to a small county to testify when several cases were going to be tried. The state's testimony in the morning case would neither help nor harm the defendant. The defense attorney would probably not even bother questioning my credentials or testimony.

Being a Southern gentleman, the defense attorney took me to lunch. The case after lunch was a totally different matter. The state's testimony would be damaging to the defendant, and the same defense attorney discredited my credentials and testimony, almost to the point of harassment. Walking out of the courtroom, I can remember the defense attorney telling me it was his job to harass me and not to take it personally. My response was, "How can I not?"

On another occasion, the defense was tearing the state's case and my testimony apart. The defense attorney was out of line with his statements. One could usually depend on the district attorney to object to such harassment. I looked over to the state's side of the table, and the district attorney was asleep. No wonder I was getting the ninth degree. I turned to the judge and told him I objected to the defense. He said I could not object. I told him the district attorney was asleep. The judge asked the assistant district attorney to wake up the district attorney.

"I Have a Dog's Head for You"

Toxicology and taxidermy are often confused. While working as a forensic toxicologist for the state of Alabama, it was not unusual for someone to call me to have an animal delivered for taxidermy. They would tell me the animal was an eight-point deer they had killed or a ten pound big-mouth bass they had just caught. I explained whom to call for taxidermy. The Auburn University School of Veterinary Medicine conducted analysis for rabies. If an animal was thought to be rabid, the head was cut off and taken for analysis. Although the Alabama Department of Forensic Sciences did the toxicological analysis on live and deceased human specimens, I suppose it seems plausible that analysis on animals could be performed there was well. Of course that was not the case. Many law enforcement officials, nevertheless, called my home or office to say, "I have a dog's head for you."

Technician Takes Fresh Surgical Specimen into Waiting Room

Olan had worked at the hospital since he was in high school. He gathered the specimens from the operating room and brought them to the laboratory. He was a histology technician, and his responsibilities included managing the Gross Room (the area where pathology specimens are transferred for pathological review and analysis) and assisting the pathologist as he cut the gross specimens.

Olan had grown up in Tuscaloosa and knew many of the patients who came to the hospital. The surgery waiting room was off the main hall between the operating rooms and the pathology department. In the process of going back and forth, a family who knew Olan stopped him and told him their daughter was having surgery that day and they were worried.

Later that the day Olan came across the specimen from the girl whose parents knew him. Olan wanted to reassure the family and thought if the family could see the seemingly benign tissue that had been removed from their daughter, they would feel better. So he took the specimen in the container of formalin to the waiting room, opened the container, and showed the tissue to the family and those with them. It went downhill from there.

Method to Increase Breast Size

A twenty-year-old white female with intense chest pain was brought to Vanderbilt Hospital emergency department by ambulance. She appeared very distressed on admission. On examination, it was determined that the pain was actually coming from her breasts. Both areolae were involved, with concentric, same-size contusions that appeared to be very painful. There were neither lacerations nor evidence of trauma. She had very little to say. Finally, after some coaxing, she said she had heard that suction pressure on the breasts would make her breasts bigger. She had placed a vacuum cleaner head on both breasts, centered on the nipples, for thirty minutes to make them larger.

Boyfriend Arrests during Intercourse

The medical examiner's office was called to assist in the investigation of an unattended death in rural Alabama. A man was found dead in his truck parked in front of a manufactured home. His girlfriend was there. It was obvious he had been dragged from the house to the truck. He was barely in the truck and in an awkward position. The girlfriend had made up a story about what had happened. When confronted by the authorities, she confessed to having moved the body. She related a more believable story.

She said both she and the decedent were married, but not to one another. They were having an affair and regularly met at the "manufactured" home (what we used to call a trailer home). They had sex as usual. Nearing what she thought was a climax, he started seizing and fell off her. Later, realizing he was dead, she became alarmed and dragged the body to his vehicle to make it look like he had died in his truck. The coroner asked her if she was not suspicious when he started seizing.

She said, "I just thought this was the way he did it. He had all those jerking movements just as he climaxed. I did not realize until later that he was dead."

IV

MEDICAL STUDENT EXPERIENCES

The real opportunity to learn medicine came with medical school. I was excited to be in medical school, but it was far more work than I had ever dreamed!

"Don't Throw Your Money Away Applying to Medical School"

I started college as a premedical student with a medical scholarship from my high school. Because my father had died and my mother was very sick and living with my grandmother, I had to work full-time during college. Needless to say, my grades were not stellar. During my third year of college, I went to see the dean of admissions at the University of Alabama School of Medicine in Birmingham. He was old and very revered. He looked at me and then looked at my grades. He saw I was working full-time and that my wife was also working full-time. He told me it cost twenty-five dollars to apply to medical school and that I should not waste my money doing do. He said I should do something useful with my money, like taking my wife out to eat, because I would never get into medical school. He also told me I would never get into the University of Alabama School of Medicine.

I left discouraged. Later, I realized he really did me a favor because that was the day I made up my mind I was going to become a doctor no matter the cost and I was going to the University of Alabama School of Medicine. Several years after that, as a senior medical student touring new students, I came across the old gentleman who had told me I would never get into medical school. I started to tell him the story but decided not to because he probably would not remember anyway.

Delivering a Black Baby to a White Woman

Obstetrics and gynecology is usually not a specialty that students go to medical school to pursue. I had a great experience doing OB-GYN and later changed my career plans to practice this specialty. I will never forget my first delivery. The patient had received her prenatal care at the medical school clinic, although I had never met her. Under the supervision of the residents that evening, I assisted with her labor. All had gone well and we had bonded. She did not have to push very long and the delivery was easy.

My patient was white and there was no question she was Caucasian. As the head of the baby came out, it had a lot of black hair and its skin seemed darker than I expected. As I dried the baby off and clamped the cord, I came to a revelation that this baby was black. How could this be? There was no one with her, and I certainly was not going to ask her why the baby was black. This was the 1970s, and I did not know of biracial marriages and women having different race babies. *Williams Obstetrics* did not have a chapter on this.

She asked, "How's the baby doing?"

I said, "Fine."

"How does she look?"

"Fine."

She asked, "When can I see the baby?"

"In a minute." I was scared for her to see it, but then I realized I had not caused it to be black. Reluctantly, I handed her the baby.

She never commented on it being black. I did not think she was colorblind. Certainly she could see it was black and she was white. I worried about it and could not sleep that night. I saw her all five days she was in the hospital, and she never commented on the baby being black.

On her last day, I went in her room to discharge her, and a tall black man was with her. She introduced him as her husband, and he thanked me for his wife's care. I was relieved.

The Best Enema in the World

The third and fourth years of medical school are the clinical years where medical students are introduced to patient care and procedures. There are many basic procedures that students learn to do, such as sewing tissue, closing incisions, inserting Foley catheters, starting IV lines, giving enemas, putting on casts, and taking out stitches.

Scott and I were assigned to the emergency department for one month. Scott's father was the program director for the hospital's family medicine residency. We learned a lot and got to do a lot because the emergency department was the busiest in Alabama.

One of the attendings asked Scott and me to give a patient an enema. A nurse brought us the enema kit and took us to the patient's room. The patient was an older gentleman who seemed glad to see us. Figure that? He said he had trouble with his bowels and had to come to the emergency room often for an enema to get his bowels to move. We had no clue how to give an enema.

The gentleman was already undressed from the waist down because he knew the drill. We did not know about the left lateral decubitus position, so we did what we knew. We pulled out the stirrups and placed him in position like we were going to do a pap smear. The patient did not tell us otherwise and continued to be appreciative. Scott opened the enema kit and pulled out the hose. It had a guard about four inches from one end indicating how far to insert. We did not know which end to put it. It seemed to us that if we were going to clean out the colon, we needed to insert about three to four feet of the tube.

We greased the hose with lubricating jelly and slid it right in, leaving only four inches hanging out of the rectum. Scott said one of us would have to hold the four inches and bend it up so the funnel to pour the water in could be attached. I secretly knew Scott really knew what to do because his father was a doctor. We attached the funnel and were ready for water, but we did not know how much to use.

We put a little soap powder into the container, filled it with warm water, poured it into the funnel, and watched it go in. The patient did not do or say anything, so we mixed up another tank and let it go in. The patient still did not say anything, so we mixed up another tank and let it fly. On the fourth tank, near the end, the gentleman said that he felt nauseous, so we stopped.

As soon as we pulled out the tube, solid and liquid stool went everywhere, spraying out like a fire hose. There was stool all over the patient, the walls, the floor, and the table. Scott and I both were covered in stool.

Scott looked over to me and said, "You know they are going to kick us out of medical school for this."

I said, "Probably so."

After about thirty minutes of blowing out feces, the man wiped himself off, got dressed, and left. I figured he would register a complaint about us and our careers would go straight down the tube into the garbage can.

The administrator of the hospital received a letter from that particular patient. The administrator said the patient had written that we had given him the best enema that he had ever received. He wanted us to be commended.

The following month, Scott and I were on another service together. One morning during rounds, Scott and I both were both paged to the emergency department. I answered the page for us. The charge nurse answered the telephone and said, "There is an older gentleman here for an enema looking for you two guys by name."

Surgeon Cannot See because of His Mask

Sterile gowns, gloves, shoe covers, and masks are required before entering an operating room. There are varieties of all of these, including masks. The surgeon I once assisted wore a fiberglass fixed mask with a single rubber band holding it in place. He liked to move it around on his face by moving his mouth and nose. During the case, he was moving the mask, and it slipped over his eyes. His mouth and nose were not covered but his eyes were; he could not see at all. Everyone's eyes were on the surgical field except for mine. I wanted to laugh, but I knew that would get me in trouble. Rather than telling anyone, he tried to move the mask down by moving his face and nose, but it would not work. So he gave in and asked the nurse anesthetist to pull it back down.

Pediatric Nurses Pose for *Playboy* Magazine

Hospitals are very busy and usually boring. Occasionally there are medical emergencies that are exciting, but not much else is.

It was fall and football season. College football is big in the South, and every year *Playboy* magazine goes to each college football conference and to each college. Girls at each school pose for revealing pictures. If selected, those pictures appear in the Southeastern Conference edition of the magazine.

Several pediatric nurses at our hospital decided to pose for *Playboy*. Few knew about this until the magazine was out on the news stands. None of the nurses posed completely naked, but all were exposed down to their waists. I am unsure how it is determined if one is going to be completely naked or partially naked. Nevertheless, they were. Word got around Tuscaloosa quickly. You could not find an issue of *Playboy* to buy within a hundred-mile radius.

This event disrupted the operation of the entire hospital, including every floor and every service. Everyone knew about it. Everyone talked about it. The residents and medical students were like hungry wolves who hung out at the pediatric nurses' station on the seventh floor, which became the most popular floor in the hospital. There was no reason to page or beep the residents or students because you knew right where they were—at the nurses' station on pediatrics. The magazine caused so much commotion that the hospital terminated all but one of the nurses who had posed.

Going to a Code 10 without Scrub Pants

Medical students always like the opportunity to learn. Getting to a Code 10 first (now a Code Blue in most hospitals) meant an opportunity to do everything: intubating the airway, securing an intravenous line, and initiating resuscitative medications. The catch was how to get to the code first. Then an idea hit us. We asked the night operators who took the code calls to call the medical students' call room before announcing the code. This could give us two minutes maximum doing the above procedures before the rest of the team arrived. It worked well.

All medical students slept together in two call rooms that were eight-by-twelve feet in size. Each room had two sets of bunk beds, sleeping four students. If there were four males, we slept in our underwear because the rooms were hot. This of course required putting on scrubs and white coats to go to the code. If women were in the room, everyone had to wear scrubs, and it was hot. One night, four guys slept in one room, in their boxers, while the girls sleep in the another call room.

At eleven p.m., the phone rang: "Code 10, fifth floor, room 543." Everyone was up and running. I put on my scrub shirt, socks, shoes, and white coat and headed down the hall. It was amazing how much cooler the hall was than the call room. Then I realized why. I had on boxers but no pants! I stopped and headed back to the call room for scrub pants. The opportunity to do any procedure that night would pass me by.

Cadillac Dealer Markets New Coupe de Ville to Students

As you near graduation from medical school, everybody wants to sell you something: life insurance, which you really need, retirement packages, and disability insurance. A group of medical students, myself included, were joined at lunch by the local Cadillac dealer, who wanted to sell us all a new car. He thought we were about to start bringing the big bucks. He was clueless, because we were so broke we could not even afford a Pepsi. We had to educate him that it would be three to eight years before anyone would have any appreciable money. He did not call back. Besides, why would a medical student want to buy a big Cadillac Coupe de Ville?

Breast Transplant

Before Health Insurance Portability and Accountability Act (HIPAA) was passed, surgery schedules were posted everywhere in the hospital, including nurses' stations. The schedule included names, ages, procedures, and diagnoses. One morning, an older surgeon was doing a double mastectomy for a benign process. Before the procedure, the surgeon and I made floor rounds ("rounds" are a teaching conference or a meeting in which clinical problems are discussed).

As we got to the seventh floor nurses' station, the unit clerk, who was the patient's sister, told the attending surgeon, "It's really a shame. Her breasts are too big, and I have none." She asked the surgeon if he could transplant her sister's breasts to her chest. She implied that anyone would then be able to tell her front from her back.

Code 10 with Unit Clerk, Maintenance Man, and Myself

I received a great clinical education as a medical student at the Tuscaloosa regional campus of the University of Alabama School of Medicine. I got to do more than most of my counterparts at the main campus in Birmingham, because there were only family medicine residents at Tuscaloosa. I got to first assist on nearly four hundred operations.

During my night on call, the hospital operator announced a Code 10 on the fourth floor. I ran there as quickly as I could, hoping to get to do a procedure. The emergency department physician was already there, so I helped as much as I could. While working on the patient, I heard the operator announce another code on the same floor at the other end of the hall. The ER attending told me to find out what was going on.

So I took off running down the hall. I passed a maintenance man working on a water fountain. He said, "Hey, I know CPR. Do you want me to help you?"

I said, "Sure. Come on."

He grabbed his tool box full of Craftsman tools and ran with me.

We both passed the nurses' station, and the only person there was the unit clerk. Everyone else was at the other code. She said, "I know CPR. Do you want my help?"

I said, "Yes, come on."

The three of us ran into the patient's room. The only equipment we had was the Craftsman toolbox. The unit secretary had a ballpoint pen.

We shook the patient and he woke—and to make a long story short, he actually did okay.

Retrieving a Vibrator from a Man's Colon

Medical students rotate through most of the hospitals in Birmingham, including the "indigent hospital." One night, a patient presented to the emergency department complaining of something in his rectum. The medical student went ahead of the team and started the workup with a history and physical.

The patient said he had placed a vibrator in his rectum and it "got away from him."

The student was perplexed and asked exactly what he meant.

The patient said, "I think it went up my rectum, and I cannot get it out."

The student was unsure what he meant but continued with the history and physical. When the student put his stethoscope on the left lower quadrant of the abdomen, it sounded like a motor running.

The student asked the patient about the noise and the patient said, "The vibrator may still be running." The student confirmed that the motor was still on. The patient said he'd used K-Y Jelly, which made the vibrator slippery and it had gotten away from him; he could not get it out.

The patient was taken to the operating room and put to sleep. The vibrator was still running and was removed by endoscopy instruments. The vibrator was switched off before being sent to pathology. It was now a "foreign body removed from the rectum."

Sometimes Babies Do Better on the First Bounce

Medical students and residents like doing procedures. Clinical years are certainly more fun than the academic years. The fun procedures on the OB-GYN Clerkship for students are deliveries, assisting at cesarean sections, performing circumcisions, and assisting at gynecologic procedures. Our service delivered about two hundred babies a month. Many of the older OB-GYN and family medicine physicians allowed medical students and residents to do their deliveries with one strict rule: residents and students could not tell anyone they did the delivery or the whole deal was off for everyone. No exceptions.

Late one night, the nurses summoned a resident and me to "help" with one of the older attending's deliveries. This meant one of us was going to get to "catch" the baby. The resident was up this time, so he scrubbed and gowned before draping the patient. The patient was already in stirrups and asleep with cyclopropane (anesthesia). The resident got ready and the nurse pressed on the fundus because the patient could not push since she was asleep.

The baby shot out and the resident tried to grab it but could not. The baby hit the floor and bounced up like a yo-yo from the elasticity of the umbilical cord. The attending said nothing and the baby appeared okay. The resident was upset and worried about being fired.

Leaving the delivery room, all the attending ever said was, "Sometimes they do better on the first bounce." It was never mentioned again.

Telephone Cord in the Urethra

During medical school, the rotation through the emergency department is an experience unto itself. I learned a lot and got to see a lot. One patient came in with a telephone cord in his urinary bladder. Now, how in this world could that ever happen? I cannot fathom the telephone company developing a system that would negotiate the male urethra and bladder to provide local and long distance service. Upon questioning, the patient actually said that he was using the cord in his urethra (which seemed even more peculiar) to enhance sexual activity. He was either bored or smarter than I was, because the sex talks I had heard at school, church, and home did not mention telephone cords. We consulted urology and they pulled out the cord with a cystoscope.

Medical Student Gets Police Escort to Hospital

Medical school clinical years at the University of Alabama School of Medicine main campus required students to go to outlying hospitals for rotations, which required driving your own vehicle to whatever hospital you were assigned to. One of my classmates was late to surgery at a distant hospital. She heard a siren, and in her rearview mirror saw a police cruiser with red and blue lights burning. It was obviously behind her so she pulled over and stopped. She looked very appropriate, dressed in nice clothes and her lab coat. Her stethoscope was around her neck. As the policeman approached her door, she rolled down the window. She asked what was wrong and the policeman said she was speeding. This came as no surprise to her.

He asked her what she was doing and where she was going. She replied that she had emergency surgery to perform at a nearby hospital; she was only hoping to avoid getting a ticket. To her amazement, the policeman never mentioned a ticket. Instead, he told her that since traffic was heavy, he would give her an emergency escort to the hospital with lights and siren. It was all she could do to keep up with him because she was in a twenty-year-old, worn out, rusted car. The officer should have been suspicious of a surgeon driving an old, beat-up car. It was kind of fun until they got closer to the hospital. She figured she would get caught. But when they got to the hospital, the officer said nothing and just waived as she ran in to assist in surgery.

"This Is a Good Boy"

Dr. David C. Sabiston Jr. was one of the most prominent surgeons ever to live. He spent most of his career at Duke University and wrote the classic *Sabiston's Textbook of Surgery*. For medical students wanting to complete a residency in surgery, Duke was usually their first choice if their credentials were sterling. One of the medical students at our school wanted to go to Duke for training. He decided that his best chance to get into a surgery residency there was to do a month's rotation at Duke, which he did.

He asked Dr. Sabiston for a letter of recommendation, which Dr. Sabiston agreed to write. The letter was simple and to the point: "This is a good boy—Sabiston." The young man was accepted to Duke for a residency in surgery.

Early in his second year, the resident was having difficulty at home because he was never there; his wife saw very little of him. So he gathered enough courage to talk with Dr. Sabiston. He told the chief what was going on. Dr. Sabiston listened intently, and then he answered, "You can always get another wife, but you can never get another surgery residency at Duke." The resident left and got back to work.

Medical Student Wears Only a Lab Coat to Code 10

During medical school, most students look for any opportunity to learn a new procedure or perform an old one. Intubating a patient at a code is a great opportunity if a medical student gets to the room before a resident or attending physician, but this requires speed. At night, getting dressed is what slowed you down. One of the female medical students came up with the idea of putting on only a lab coat before speeding to the code. She slept naked so the lab coat was all she had on at codes. Her apparel created quite a stir!

V

RESIDENCY TRAINING IN PATHOLOGY AND OB-GYN

During residency training, new interns learn about the real practice of medicine and build on that knowledge each year. Instead of paying tuition, interns actually get paid a salary. It was hectic, stressful, long hours, sometimes humiliating, occasionally empowering, and oftentimes demanding. Attendings wanted you to go home and read, but sometimes it was all you could do to hold your head up. Overall, it was a great experience.

Senior Resident Explains to Family about Cancer

A family from rural Alabama had brought their father to University Hospital for evaluation of a possible cancer. After talking with the patient in the intensive care unit, the medical team came to the waiting room to speak with the family. The team consisted of the attending surgeon, the chief resident, a senior resident, two interns, and four medical students. Everyone was quiet as the attending surgeon spoke to the family. He told them that their father had a poorly differentiated, metastatic, squamous cell carcinoma invading the pterygium and penetrating the capsule. You could tell by their faces they had no idea what he was talking about. There was a far-off look in their eyes.

Being from rural Alabama himself, the senior resident stepped up and asked the attending surgeon if he could explain to the family what the attending had just said. He turned to the family, and in his

Southern drawl said, "Your daddy has cancer. It's the eating kind and it's done commenced to eat."

They said, "Oh, we understand what you mean. Thank you."

Baby Delivered with a Vacuum Cleaner

Women deliver babies either vaginally or by cesarean section. Occasionally, vaginal deliveries require the use of instruments such as forceps or vacuum extractors. The current patient had to have her baby delivered by a vacuum extractor. This was explained to her, which she seemed to understand. However, when she returned for her postpartum checkup, she announced that her baby had been delivered by a vacuum cleaner. We never could get her to understand the difference.

"Nosmoking"

Not all laboring women in the 1970s and '80s used epidural anesthesia. Many still labored and delivered with intravenous narcotics and sedation. One of my patients using narcotics and sedation progressed to the time of delivery. We moved her to the delivery room and she pushed out a seven pound healthy boy without complications. I have always asked parents what they plan to name their children. Today, with ultrasounds during prenatal care, most know the sex of the baby, have named the baby, have purchased sex-appropriate clothes, and have painted the nursery.

Before ultrasound, mothers had to wait until delivery to learn their baby's gender. Many thought about names for a few days before naming the baby. I always suggested my favorites for them to consider: "Daniel" or "Danielle."

This patient did not have a name for her baby and wanted to think about it. On postpartum day, I went in to see her. She told me she had come up with a name. She said she named her little boy "Nosmoking." I asked her how she came up with that name. She said she had received it in a vision as she went into the delivery room. She said the name was in large, bright-red letters and she knew it was the right name. I told her she had seen the "no smoking" sign outside the delivery room and that it meant not to smoke inside the delivery room. The baby was still named "Nosmoking."

Capitol Rotunda

The very same scenario happened the same day in labor and delivery. A patient heard a voice telling her what to name her baby as she was carried into the delivery room. She named her baby "Capitol Rotunda." Actually, the voice was that of the television. A dignitary was lying in state in the capitol rotunda in Washington, DC. The child was still named "Capitol Rotunda."

Caught in the Elevator at University Hospital

One Saturday, I was on "floater call" for OB-GYN as a third-year resident at University Hospital. I floated between University Hospital and the indigent hospital three blocks down the street. I covered GYN and backed up the residents covering OB at both places. University Hospital had eighteen floors, and the resident call rooms were on the seventeenth floor. Things were quiet, so I decided to get some sleep. A few minutes into a nap, I was paged stat to labor and delivery downstairs on the fifth floor at University Hospital. I got dressed, ran to the elevator, and got in. The elevator went a couple of floors and then stopped. There was an emergency phone on the elevator, so I picked it up and called for help.

The hospital operator called the elevator company. A repair crew could not come until Monday morning, but this was Saturday night. I told the operator that I needed out tonight. I asked her to call labor and delivery and tell them I was trapped in the elevator. She said she would call maintenance for help.

About thirty minutes later, a maintenance crew pried the door open about one foot so I could see them but could not get out. I was trapped between floors. The crew told me that in order for me to get out, I would have to crawl out of the elevator into the adjacent elevator. I said, "Okay."

The maintenance men explained to me how to remove a panel on the wall of the elevator, allowing access to the shaft. The men told me not to look down because I was seventeen floors up and it was a straight drop down. I had to squeeze between the greasy elevator cables and walk on steel beams.

"Don't look down," they said.

Unfortunately, I looked down and should not have. Now I was dizzy. I squeezed through the cables and got grease all over me.

The men had opened the hatch to the other elevator, and I got in. I went to the delivery room, but the delivery was over. I was covered with black grease. They all asked, "What happened to you?"

I said, "I got stuck in the elevator."

Someone Calls Every Night Threatening to Jump off a Building

Every night, someone called labor and delivery and threatened to jump off the top floor of the hospital. The resident working labor and delivery would spend thirty minutes talking to this person and persuading him or her not to jump. This went on most nights for about six months.

One night when we were very busy, we heard from the same caller with the usual story we'd heard every night. One of the chief residents had fielded the call and decided enough was enough. The chief resident said, "Jump, jump, jump!" No one ever called back again. We checked the newspapers for weeks to see if someone had jumped off a building but never found anything.

Patient in the Emergency Room with "Cervical Cancer"

A resident on call at night could expect to see anything and everything. One evening, I was paged to the indigent hospital to see a patient in the emergency department diagnosed with cervical cancer. I was told she would need to be admitted to the hospital for a radical hysterectomy. She had been seen by an attending physician.

On the way to the emergency department, I rehearsed in my mind the staging for cervical cancer and the various treatments. When I got there, I went in to talk to the patient, who at this point was distraught and appropriately so, after receiving a diagnosis of cervical cancer. After talking to her, I asked if I could examine her. She agreed.

I carefully slipped in the speculum, trying not to disturb anything and certainly not stir up bleeding. Then I saw a white solid mass filling the top of the vagina. I saw no bleeding. For some reason, the mass did not look right. It was too uniform and there was no necrosis. I took a pair of ring forceps and touched it. There was no bleeding and it felt spongy. Then I pulled on it and it started coming out. It was a tampon packed in there. It smelled awful because it had been in there a long time, but there was no cancer. The patient was relieved. The attending was very upset.

Internal Medicine Resident Examining the Vagina

After the emergency department physician assesses a patient, the pertinent service is called to complete the care of the patient in what is called a consultation. On one occasion, the gynecology service were consulted for a vaginitis, which is a little unusual, but I headed to the emergency department. Upon arriving, I checked the patient's chart. The ER attending physician said the internal medicine resident on the service was still looking at the vaginitis, but we could go in and see the patient. I opened the door. What I saw I had never seen before nor since. I could not believe my eyes.

The internal medicine resident was indeed looking at the inside of the vagina. However, instead of using a vaginal speculum with a light, he was looking into the vagina with an otoscope (a device used to examine the ears). He had most of the otoscope inside the vagina with his left eye on the lens, making his entire face about an inch from the perineal skin.

I said, "Can you see anything?"

He said he could see everything.

I told him his otoscope would never be the same. I asked him if he had ever heard of a vaginal speculum, and he nodded to the affirmative.

I said, "You're kind of close, aren't you?" I told him I needed to look but would use a vaginal speculum.

Body Transported through Cafeteria

University Hospital in Birmingham, Alabama, is a one-thousand-bed teaching hospital and quaternary referral center for Alabama. The cafeteria is located in the middle of the hospital, with many of the beds in the towers on one side and Hillman Clinic and specialty clinics on the other.

Patients are not usually carried through the cafeteria. One patient transporter, however, chose to carry a patient in a wheelchair through the cafeteria. The patient was sick, and to spare everyone from seeing him, he covered his head with a sheet. For some reason, several hospital employees thought the patient was dead and being carried through the cafeteria to the morgue. It is difficult enough to get a dead body to sit in a wheelchair, much less risk it falling out onto the floor. Dead bodies are typically covered and carried to the morgue on stretchers, using the service elevators.

Unfortunately, a complaint about the "dead" patient in the cafeteria reached administration, and the department of pathology was reprimanded for carrying a dead body through the cafeteria. It took some investigative work to sort out what happened.

Grandmother Breast-Feeds Baby

During residency training, a pregnant sixteen-year-old was transferred to labor and delivery at University Hospital from rural Alabama with severe preeclampsia. She was accompanied by her mother, who stayed with her the entire hospital course. The teenager died after serious complications of the delivery. The grandmother took the baby to raise. A few months later, I saw the grandmother with the baby at Children's Hospital. To my amazement, the grandmother was breast-feeding the baby. I asked her how she was able to breast-feed, and she said she wanted to and her milk came down. She had been able to make enough milk to satisfy the baby.

Surgery Resident Fakes Seizure in Operating Room

For a variety of reasons, most residents after the internship year moonlight to increase their income, pay off school loans, buy a house, etc. They moonlight at night during the week and on weekends. The money is especially helpful for residents with families and those residents who need a little spending money. Moonlighting comes with a price, however, because residents are usually tired after moonlighting but still have to do their regular job as a resident with its demands, long hours, and call.

One of the surgery residents, John, had the misfortune of moonlighting and not sleeping all night. During the first case the next morning, he fell asleep at the operating table. To make things worse, he grabbed the surgical drapes, pulling them off the patient and emptying the instrument tray onto the floor. The noise woke him just before he hit the floor, and he realized what was going on. So he kept his eyes closed and jerked his arms and legs like he was having a seizure. One of the other residents immediately picked up on what was going on. He told the attending surgeon that John had seizures and did this all the time and would be okay. John was not reprimanded.

Resident Could Not Tell If Patient Was Dead

In teaching hospitals, it is the interns who are called to pronounce a patient dead, speak with the family, and write a death note. Medical students have no exposure to this and it is, thereby, a new experience for new interns. What most interns do not appreciate is that by the time the house staff is called, the nurse has determined that the patient is dead, the family has been told, and the family members are deciding on a funeral home and have usually left the hospital. The job of the intern just makes all this formal.

An intern just could not tell if the patient was dead. He often did lab work, which was of no help. He ordered EKGs and they were flat line. I believe he worried the patient was comatose with hard-to-detect vital signs. Even with the nurse's coaxing, it was a struggle to make the decision that this patient had "passed on."

Tired Surgery Residents Talk to the Chief about Workload

The chief of surgery at the University Hospital in Birmingham was the most prominent general and thoracic surgeon of his time. Most medical students wanting to match in a surgery residency wanted to train with him. Training at University Hospital opened doors that otherwise would be closed when it came to looking for a job. Unfortunately, that great training came with a great price, sacrificing almost everything else in life; nothing was spared.

An intern and second-year resident found enough courage to talk to the chief of surgery. They were gracious and proper and so was he. They told him they thought they were having to work too much. The chief's face did not change as he turned around to the table behind his desk and dialed a phone number. The house staff could not hear his voice. After several minutes he hung up and turned back around to the intern and resident.

He told the two he could help them and they smiled. He told them he had gotten both of them jobs at the Alabama Theater taking up tickets. They needed to be there at five p.m. dressed in tuxedos. The intern and resident were speechless, and they ran out of the chief of surgery's office and never mentioned hard work again; neither did the chief.

Resident Eats Food Directly from Tray instead of a Plate

Medical students and residents can be some of the hungriest people in the hospital. As a general rule, if food is left uneaten, the house staff will eat it. Anything is fair game. Whether it is the long hours and work, or the lack of money, or both, residents and medical students can eat large amounts of food. One resident I worked with used two plates on his tray in the physician's cafeteria, known as the "GI Lab." Two plates were still not enough, so the cafeteria staff suggested this resident allow them to put his food directly on the tray and to just forget the plates. This worked out well for him and for the cafeteria staff, but it looked strange for food to be piled high on just the tray.

Naked Obstetric Patient Runs down the Hall

Patients of all walks of life receive their care in the indigent health-care system. Those who are pregnant go to the local health department for obstetric care and then deliver at the indigent hospital. One high-risk patient who had chronic hypertension quit taking her six antihypertensive medications despite the warning by her mother, who was a registered nurse. The patient presented to labor and delivery with shortness of breath. We were uncertain how high her blood pressure was because the blood pressure monitor was thumping at the top of the spygmomaneter at 300mm Hg systolic and 160mm Hg diastolic (300/160). During the assessment by the nurse, the pregnant patient pulled off all her clothes, belted out of the room, and ran down the hall. We could not catch her, so we called security, and eventually she was caught. She was in florid pulmonary edema (an abnormal buildup of fluid in the air sacs of the lungs), requiring intravenous lasix and intubation. In retrospect, I suspect she was short of breath and thought taking off her clothes and running down the hall might help.

Patient Uses Genitalia to Stop Oscillating Fan

Interns in most specialties rotate through the emergency department. All kinds of patients and conditions present to the emergency department to be treated. One Saturday evening, a young man covered with blood presented to the department.

Upon questioning, he said he had used his penis to stop an oscillating fan.

The intern said, "This is the craziest story I have ever heard."

The patient said, "Wait and hear my side of the story. It was an eight-inch plastic fan from Sears. I bragged to my girlfriend that I could stop it with my penis."

I asked him what happened, and he said the fan had chopped up his penis. He took off the towel covering his genitalia. Sure enough, the penis looked like it had been through a meat grinder. The urology service was consulted to try to repair it. I was sure it would never be the same again.

Interns Called to Break Up Sexual Intercourse

One of the duties of interns is to go into patient rooms and stop them from having sexual intercourse. I suppose there is an unwritten rule that patients should not have sex in the hospital, but there are many reasons people have sex in the hospital. First, the hospital is a different place where most people have not tried to have sex before. Second, there is the excitement that you might get caught. Third, patients may have run out of things to talk about. Fourth, as a patient, you are clean (most people clean up before coming to the hospital). Fifth, you might miss having sex at home and do not want to miss a night. Sixth, you make amends for something you have done wrong, and sex is part of the making up. Seventh, the hospital gown looks "sexy." Eighth, you just want to have sex, and this is as good a place as any.

As an intern, do you knock on the door or burst right in, hoping to catch the couple in the act? Do you knock on the door and say, "What are y'all doing? Are you busy? Is anyone at home?" Most of the time, you just go in and ask them to please quit or wait until they get home.

Dirty Penis Syndrome

During residency training at the university, grand rounds were presented each week at noon by one of the house staff. Grand rounds were attended by the chairman, faculty, staff, fellows, residents, medical students from OB-GYN, as well faculty and house staff from other specialties such as pathology, surgery, urology, and anesthesiology. Each resident was responsible for a presentation, including overhead slides, handouts, references, and pathology slides.

Karen had the idea that sexually transmitted diseases in women came from men who did not wash their hands. Men are taught from early boyhood to wash their hands after urinating. Men handled all kinds of things all day and contaminated their penis with all manner of infections. Then they urinate by holding their penis with their dirty hands. They go home at night and have intercourse with their wives with a dirty, contaminated penis, causing infections.

Her conclusion was that men should was their hands *before urinating* rather than afterward to keep their penis clean. This would reduce infections in women. Karen presented this theory as grand rounds and entitled it as the "Dirty Penis Syndrome"—except "penis" was not the word used. It created quite a stir and some interesting discussion at grand rounds.

Male Presents to the ER with a Picture Tube in His Rectum

More curious things happen in the emergency department than any other area in the hospital. Patients present with the strangest stories, many of which are true. A twenty-five-year-old male presented to the ER with a complaint that a television picture was in his rectum, and he could not get it out. A flat and upright X-ray of the abdomen showed a television picture tube in the descending colon. The surgery service was consulted, and an intern interviewed the patient. The patient complained that he'd needed to take a bath. And, completely unbeknownst to him, he said, a television picture tube was sitting in the tub, which was filled with water. He did not notice the tube, and as he sat in the water, the tube went right up his rectum. Imagine that! My question was why a picture tube would be in the tub anyway. It is interesting that as he sat down in the water, the picture tube was perfectly lined up with his rectum and slid right in.

A digital examination could not identify the picture tube, so the patient was told he needed to go to surgery to have the tube removed. He would be sedated and the surgery service would try to get the tube out endoscopically. If that failed, he would have an open laparotomy. The patient then confessed that he was using the picture tube in his rectum. He had greased his rectum with KY Jelly so the tube would slide in. Because his hands were slippery, the tube got away from him and he could not retrieve it. So he came to the hospital. I think if I was in his position, I would have gone to a hospital in Canada where no one knew me.

A few weeks later another man came to the ER with a similar complaint. He had been using a mustard jar in his rectum and it got away from him. He had to go to the operating room for retrieval under general anesthesia. Simpson obstetrics forceps were used to retrieve the jar.

Surgery Resident Licks End of Suture

Cardiac surgery at the University of Alabama in Birmingham is a big event because patients from all over the world come to UAB to have their chests cracked open. Most of the work is done by cardiac surgery fellows, but on occasion, surgery residents get to scrub in—and on rarer occasions, even medical students. On one particular occasion, the attending surgeon left the case for the fellows to close. A resident was asked to close the incision. Although "pop off" and "non pop off" needles were in widespread use in medicine at the time, the sutures to close with on this case required manually threading permanent needles. Threading the suture was hard for the resident because this type of needle was rarely used.

Without thinking, the resident pulled up his mask and licked the suture so it would slide into the eye of the needle. This stopped the case . . .

Morbidly Obese Patient Kicks Senior Resident off the Bed

J. C. was one of the best senior residents. He always helped the junior residents and interns as much as possible, and he was a great teacher. One night at the indigent hospital in Birmingham, he decided to help manage the large number of patients in labor. One of the patients was a young woman who was morbidly obese and very difficult to deal with. No one had been successful in checking her cervix because she would not let them; it was a difficult examination under the best of circumstances.

J. C. decided to show the lower level house staff how to manage this type of situation. He coaxed the patient into the dorsal lithotomy position and started inserting two fingers into her vagina. The patient, who weighed in excess of four hundred pounds, put her foot on his chest, screamed, and catapulted him off the bed, through the air, and onto the floor.

J. C. was quite stunned as he got up. He turned to the patient and said, "You don't want to be ugly to the person who controls your pain medicine." He then walked into the hall and with his deep bass voice shouted to the nursing station, "No pain medicine for room number 2!"

Psychiatric Patient Swallows Resident's Sunglasses

The hospital where I completed my OB-GYN residency was an eight-hundred-bed teaching hospital. The entire seventh floor was for psychiatry only. Residents rarely went to this floor, except to see a consultation. The seventh floor was definitely not a place to "hang out." The attending physician provided us with a consultation for us to work up for the great enigma of pelvic pain, one of the most difficult diagnostic challenges in gynecology. Pelvic pain in a mental patient would be even more challenging.

The chief resident, an intern, and I headed to the seventh floor. There was a patient who had eaten everything in sight: nails, ballpoint pens, silver coins, etc. Radiographs looked like everything was in her stomach except the kitchen sink. She'd had multiple previous surgeries to remove many items from her stomach.

So we went to see this patient with pelvic pain. Taking the patient's history was difficult, and the examination was worse. As the chief resident leaned over to examine the patient, the patient grabbed his expensive sunglasses out of the pocket of his white coat and swallowed them. The chief ranted and raved about losing his expensive sunglasses. We left the floor after presenting to the attending.

We had forgotten about the sunglasses because we were so busy. About a week later, the chief resident was paged to the seventh floor. As he answered the page, the nurse on the other end replied: "We've got your sunglasses."

Resident Becomes Mr. Mom

Society and physicians themselves feel that doctors have the most difficult jobs in life. The problems they deal with can be perplexing. Physicians work long hours and often all night. During residency training, I had an eye-opening experience. My wife went on a business trip to another state. I had four weeks' vacation, and I agreed to use one week to keep our newborn baby, three-year-old, and four-year-old while she was away. I thought this would be a piece of cake and a good, restful week for a hardworking resident. I would normally have had a full workweek and three nights of call. I had no clue that I was exchanging that for seven days and nights, twenty-four hours a day.

Day one, they all cried for their mother. I extinguished this by allowing the kids to stay up as long as they wanted and eat whatever they wished. Walking around picking up toys, flushing commodes, gathering clothes to wash, bathing kids and a baby, and changing diapers seemed more demanding than a radical hysterectomy and certainly less fun. By day three, no one liked my cooking. To save time, I decided to let the three- and four-year-old bathe themselves.

I sent the four-year-old to turn on the water in the tub in the children's bathroom, which was upstairs. She did and came downstairs to watch a cartoon show on television. All was well until I thought I heard water running, then I didn't, then I did, and then it stopped, so I did not worry.

I got up to go to the kitchen when I noticed water was flowing down the stairs—in fact, pouring down the stairs. I asked the four-year-old if she turned the water off in the tub and she said, "Daddy, you did not tell me to do that!"

I suspected the problem to be in the kids' bathroom. It was. The tub was overflowing, filling the bathroom, the hall, and flowing down the stairs. Carpets everywhere were wet. I cut the water off and started the clean up. Unfortunately, ServPro (for damage restoration) had not been created yet.

Rope Hanging Out of the Vagina

Telephone calls from OB-GYN patients at Carraway Methodist Medical Center were forwarded to labor and delivery and given to the junior or senior resident on call. It did not matter who the calls were from; they might be private patients or teaching clinic patients.

One of the chief residents took one of the calls. A man said his wife's water had broken and that a rope was hanging out of his wife's vagina. "The rope beats like your heart," the man said.

The chief resident, realizing the man was describing a prolapsed cord, jumped out of his chair and told the man to bring his wife to the hospital as soon as he could. The phone call turned out to be prank by some of the junior residents, who were playing jokes on the chief that night. The prank did not go so well with the chief.

Physician by Day, Fireman by Night

One night, my five-year-old son asked if we could cook hamburgers on the grill. So, why not? I had just gotten in from the hospital, and the idea sounded good. I told him we would get the fire started, I would change clothes, and then he could help me grill the burgers. It was getting dark, so I knew we needed to hurry. We put the charcoal on the grill and lit it. I told him to stay away from the fire so he would not get hurt because the fire would burn him. I went inside to change clothes.

No sooner than I had gotten my clothes off and down to my underwear than I noticed it seemed very bright outside, which was impossible because it had been nearly dark. I walked over to the window and could not believe what I saw. My son had taken a cardboard cylinder, the kind wrapping paper came on, and put it in the now-blazing fire, making a torch. He then used the torch to set every bush and scrub in our backyard on fire. It was as bright as day outside. I ran out and got the garden hose, extinguishing the fires before the neighbors could call the fire department.

By now my other children and their mother were outside. I told them what had happened. I told my son I was going to whip him.

My wife said, "Not so quick! I remember you setting West End Elementary School on fire when you were young. It's probably genetic."

Surgery Residents Get Headlights

The general surgery residency program at Carraway Methodist Medical Center in Birmingham, Alabama, was a well-respected, time-honored general surgery residency where many of the practicing general surgeons in Alabama had trained over the years. Many graduates have gone on to pursue surgical subspecialties. One of the up and coming instruments to allow surgeons to see better at the operating table was headlights. So the surgery residents asked medical education and the surgery department to get headlights for the residents to use when they were operating. This never materialized. To make a point, the residents used duct tape to secure "D cell" flashlights to the top of their scrub caps. The flashlights were not very effective but quite amusing and made the point.

New Intern "Cardioverts" His Head

For decades, advanced cardiovascular life support (ACLS) has been part of orientation for new interns, and every specialty participated. One particular morning, we were defibrillating mannequins. At lunch, we broke for an hour. Several of the interns wandered into the cardiopulmonary resuscitation area, but no one realized the defibrillators were still fully charged. One intern decided to play with a defibrillator, placed the paddles on either side of his head, and fired away. Three hundred joules of electrical current went through his head, melting his metal glasses and knocking him onto the floor. It took a minute for the other interns to realize what had happened. The intern survived but had significant burns. After that, we were very careful when using the defibrillators.

Postpartum Magnesium Patient in Call Bed

Obstetric call at the county's indigent hospital could be brutal. One evening, we had done twenty-one deliveries by a third-year resident, two interns, and two medical students supervised by the chief resident. The medical students did the vaginal deliveries, the interns the more complicated deliveries, the third-year resident the cesarean sections, and the chief resident supervised. All the labor rooms were filled. Patients filled the recovery room and spilled into the hallways.

The deliveries were finally completed, so I decided to try to get some sleep. I went to the call room to find a patient in my call room bed. I went to the nursing desk and inquired why, and the nurses responded there was nowhere else to put the patient.

No sleep for me that night!

Psychiatry Resident Has Sex with Patient

A patient was hospitalized where I completed a residency in obstetrics and gynecology. Psychiatry was consulted because the patient was distraught about marital issues at home. A male psychiatry resident, after interviewing the patient, determined the patient needed intimacy. After holding her, kissing began, leading to sexual intercourse in the hospital bed. The resident was caught, and during the disciplinary hearing, he responded that he determined the patient needed sex to feel better.

Female Resident Asks to Borrow a Pair of My Underwear

Karen, a fellow resident, and I were assigned to the indigent hospital for a twenty-four-hour shift. She was wonderful. Karen performed a complicated vaginal delivery accompanied by a massive hemorrhage. The patient lost a lot of blood, most of which ended up on Karen. Bleeding had been stopped and the patient stabilized, but Karen was soaked.

Leaving the delivery room, she asked, "Can I borrow a pair of your underwear?"

I said, "For what?"

She said, "To wear."

I said, "We wear different sizes, and I only have one pair."

"Not a Doctor; He Works in the Boiler Room"

In "the old days," OB-GYN training included general surgery training and emergency medicine. Saturday nights usually meant a lot of tissue sewing in the emergency department on patients who were drunk. Many of these patients were so inebriated they did not even require local anesthesia to put in sutures. But drunk patients can be hard to deal with, even combative, so several security officers were always in the emergency areas.

While sewing up several large lacerations on the back of a patient, he asked who was sewing him up. Before I could respond, the security officer told the patient I was not a doctor and that I worked in the boiler room as a maintenance man and had learned how to sew tissue. When the ER was busy, I was often called to help sew patients. I could never convince the patient that the guard was teasing and that I really was a doctor.

Ultrasounding "Patient" outside the Emergency Department

My fellow resident Karen and I were on at University Hospital obstetrics call one night. She paged me and asked me to bring the ultrasound machine from labor and delivery to the emergency department. We did this regularly so we could do our own ultrasounds because it saved a lot of time.

As I got to the emergency department, I asked Karen where to bring the ultrasound machine. She was a little sheepish and said we were going to do an ultrasound outside on the sidewalk. I have never done an ultrasound outside, and it did not seem like a good idea. I thought she was kidding, but she walked out to the ambulance ramp. There was her car, pulling a horse trailer.

I said, "What's up?"

She said, "We're going to ultrasound my pregnant horse." (This was worse than the underwear scheme.) I told her if we got caught (and how could we manage not to?), we would be terminated. I envisioned having to tell my wife that I was no longer in residency but was now sacking groceries at Piggly Wiggly. I did not help ultrasound the horse.

Unusual Ultrasound Pictures

Ultrasound was first used in medicine around 1980 and was soon available widespread. Most OB-GYN residents learned how to perform basic ultrasonography. Our hospital had a small portable sonar machine in labor and delivery for a "quick look." My youngest daughter had a small set of plastic animal templates that she used to trace animals. Looking at them, I suspected the templates would fit on the screen of the portable sonar in labor and delivery. So I took a few templates with me to work.

Having no idea what to expect, patients would often ask to see what their baby looked like. We would put one of the templates on the sonar screen before switching the machine on. When it was turned on, a white field normally appeared, but with a template on it, an outline of an animal was apparent. The shock on their face was priceless.

The resident would say, "Here is your baby—it is so cute."

The patient would then say it looked like a German shepherd or an alligator. Then they got to see the real thing and were relieved.

Clinic Patients Converted to Breech for Experience

The American College of Obstetricians and Gynecologist announced this past year that the appropriate management of a pregnant patient in labor with a breech presentation is a cesarean section. This has not always been the case. Many breech presentations have, in the past, been delivered vaginally. Breech presentations are not common, but physicians who deliver babies need to know how to manage them.

In the old days, the program director at our residency believed competency delivering breech babies was necessary. So he took clinic patients who were headfirst and performed external version, converting them to breech presentations so the residents could have ample practice with breech births. That would be considered inappropriate and unacceptable today.

OB-GYN Residents Perform Neurosurgery

Like most OB-GYN residencies, we had rotations in general surgery. Night call included covering all surgical subspecialties. A first- and a second-year OB-GYN resident were on call when a patient with a subdural hematoma arrived by ambulance in the emergency department. One resident stabilized the patient while the other called the attending neurosurgeon on call.

The surgeon said, "I'm on my way. Go ahead and get the patient asleep. My nurse will show you how to do a bur hole. By then I will be there for the good part."

When the anesthesiologist got there, he said, "When did you boys get your neurosurgery boards?"

He knew neither had received any neurosurgery training. When the attending neurosurgeon got there, he was drunk and could not operate. So the nurse showed the OB-GYN residents how to perform the surgery and then helped them close. Luckily the patient did well.

Gynecologic Surgery Patient with Chest Pain during Intercourse

Residency training provided new experiences every day. Residents had surgery and made rounds with the attendings every morning. Residents assigned to attendings made pre-rounds by themselves and then rounded with their attendings.

In medicine, you never can predict what a patient might say. Several residents, the chief resident, and two medical students were rounding with the OB-GYN department chairman. He was prim and proper and a Southern gentleman. While talking with a patient, she said, "During intercourse, I have chest pain."

The chairman, without batting an eye, immediately responded, "It just goes to show that your husband is doing a good job!"

Penis Goes Up in Smoke

In the mid-1980s, a new medical issue in OB-GYN emerged—the human papillomavirus (HPV). We began seeing abnormal pap smears and genital warts. Many of these patients received laser ablation of lesions in the GYN clinic under local anesthesia.

A patient was receiving a laser vaporization of the cervix under local anesthesia. Her husband accompanied her to the visit and asked many questions. The attending answered his questions as the attending lasered the patient. The husband casually mentioned that he had warts on his penis. The attending encouraged him to seek treatment from his physician. The husband asked the attending to treat him too. The attending agreed and told the husband to pull down his pants as they stood there by his wife, which he did. The husband's penis was covered with warts.

The attending began lasering the husband's penis without anesthesia. As the husband saw his penis going up in smoke, his eyes rolled back into his head and he fainted. He did not return with his wife for her next treatment.

"I Am Going to Whip Your #%&*! When We Get Home"

Dr. Thomas Mendenhall Bouleware arrived at Carraway Methodist Medical Center in 1929 to be the first board-certified obstetrician in Alabama. Dr. Bouleware practiced obstetrics for forty-nine years. He was an oral examiner for the American Board of Obstetrics and Gynecology and gave examinations at Carraway Methodist Medical Center in Birmingham for years. Later, he started an obstetrics and gynecology residency at the hospital. To my knowledge, he was sued only once.

Dr. Bouleware lived next door to a prominent plaintiff attorney. They were longtime friends and raised their children together. The attorney had a son who practiced law with his father. Later in his career, Dr. Bouleware was sued by the son, his next-door neighbor.

As the story goes, Dr. Bouleware was on the witness stand defending himself. The son's questioning bordered on harassment. Dr. Bouleware stopping talking to the jury, turned to the attorney son, and said, "When we get home, I am going to whip your #%&*!" This, of course, created chaos and laughter in the courtroom. The jury delivered a verdict in favor of Dr. Bouleware. Dr. Bouleware was never sued again.

A Snack during Cardiovascular Surgery

Many operations in teaching hospitals can last a long time, including, for example, pelvic exenteration, cardiac bypass surgery, and complicated neurosurgery cases. The problems associated with long operations are hunger, thirst, needing to go to the restroom, pain from standing or bending, and fatigue from holding retractors. Eating a meal before surgery helps, as does having adequate fluid intake.

One senior surgery resident on the cardiovascular service devised a way to get a snack during a long case. He used a mask that had a bill-like front, where he put corn chips. All went well until he coughed during a case, blowing corn chips into the open pericardial cavity. The resident was convinced he would be thrown out of the residency, but he was not.

Unusual Delivery with Incense Burning and Husband Naked

Most labors and deliveries are fairly typical. The patient is either induced or determined to be in labor and admitted. Laboratory studies are obtained, permits signed, and epidural anesthesia is instituted at the appointed time. A small group of patients and husbands develop what is called an individual birth plan. They design their birthing experience, and the obstetrician determines how much is feasible, safe, and reasonable. For instance, I had a patient who wanted the family pet in the delivery because "it would be a good experience for him." My question was whether the dog really cared.

Another couple designed their birth plan and the OB-GYN department chair was on call for obstetrics when the patient arrived in labor. The couple went over the birth plan with the chairman, who was generally open-minded. He was okay with beads being strung up everywhere and incense burning but was a little uncomfortable with the husband being completely naked, lying in bed with his laboring wife. The baby was delivered and everything went well.

But when the husband wanted to eat the placenta, the chair refused. He said, "We have to draw the line somewhere. No."

Open Reduction Internal Fixation of Dog's Hip

Dr. Ben Myers was an orthopedic legend for many years at Carraway Methodist Medical Center in Birmingham. Patients came from all over the Southern United States to see Dr. Myers. The men's surgery dressing room was located on the third floor of the hospital, with large windows overlooking Carraway Boulevard and Twenty-Sixth Street North. A dog wandered out into the busy street and was hit by a car. Seeing what had happened, Dr. Myers sent two male attendants, then called "orderlies," from the operating room to pick up the dog from the street and bring it to the operating room. Dr. Myers examined it and determined it needed surgery to repair a broken hip.

Sometimes surgeons and anesthesiologists mix just like water and oil. I wish I could have been there when Dr. Myers told the anesthesiologist on call that he needed to put a dog to sleep in the main operating room. Dr. Myers won the battle and the dog had surgery and was kept until it healed.

Delivery of Huge Fecalith with Simpson Forceps

An obstetric patient showed up in the emergency department complaining of no bowel movement. She was approximately thirty-two weeks' gestational age but was not receiving any prenatal care. She measured thirty-two weeks, and fetal heart tones were present at 150 beats per minute. The abdomen was soft with decreased bowel sounds. Vaginal examination was precluded by a mass completely obscuring the vagina. The vagina "stopped" about five centimeters in. Rectal examination revealed a concrete-like mass filling the canal. She said she had not had a bowel movement since Thanksgiving; it was now February 15. Vaginal delivery would have been completely impossible. Later she admitted to being a prostitute with a "subspecialty interest" in anal intercourse.

The resident on call tried to remove the impaction for about three hours. The stool was rock hard and the smell was atrocious. Only liquid stool would pass around the fecalith. One of the problems with digging for hours is that despite a long hot shower and clean scrubs, you still smelled like feces. Sometimes your own family will not let you into the house. I am sure all this digging was unpleasant for the patient as well.

The residents dug in four-hour shifts. The next major medical advance and the next step for the patient was placing epidural anesthesia, as if for labor and delivery. The level was sufficient, the rectum could be better dilated, and there was great pain relief for the patient.

We started digging in four-hour shifts twice a day for five days. On Friday, the chief resident decided to perform a reverse episiotomy and deliver the fecalith with Simpson obstetrical forceps. It worked. The patient went home the next day with instructions to follow up at the indigent clinic, but she did not show up.

Eight weeks later, she showed up in active labor. Sure enough, another fecalith!

Dizziness Managed by Surgery Resident

Residents at another teaching hospital were assigned primary-care patients to care for during their entire residency. It did not matter what specialty their residency was or what service they were on, they had to care for their primary-care patients. One surgery resident had a middle-aged female patient who always came to the emergency department complaining of dizziness. Nothing could ever be found to explain the dizziness. Besides, she looked perfectly fine and probably felt better than the resident.

So the resident decided to demonstrate to her what he thought her dizziness was like. He asked her to sit upright on the examination table. He mixed several hundred ccs of ice water. He took a 60cc syringe, attached a catheter to it, and put the free end into her ear canal. He quickly infused 100ccs of ice-cold water into her ear canal.

She fell onto the floor with nystagmus (voluntary or involuntary eye movements), nausea, and vomiting. While she was rolling around on the floor, the resident told her what she was experiencing was dizziness, and if this happened to her again, she needed to come to the emergency department. If she did not experience these symptoms, she did not need to come to the hospital. The resident was not dismissed but was disciplined severely.

Resident Wears Boy Scout Hat to Cut Surgical Specimens

Dr. Long was a resident in pathology. Growing up, he had also been a Boy Scout. Pathology residents spend a significant amount of time in surgical pathology. The mornings are spent reading the slides from the day before. The afternoons are spent cutting the fresh specimens sent from surgery. Dr. Long wore his old Boy Scout hat while cutting specimens in the afternoon. He kept the hat on the shelf just above where he cut specimens. As he sat down each afternoon, he pulled the hat off the shelf and flipped it right onto his head. He did this every day.

The other residents, observing this pattern, decided to add some spice to the afternoons. They slipped a fresh, bloody placenta into Dr. Long's hat. Dr. Long arrived as usual, pulled the hat off the shelf, and flipped it onto his head. The fresh placenta slid down his face onto his freshly starched Brooks Brothers shirt. The hat was never the same.

Seeing Eye Dog Growls at OB-GYN

Assistance dogs are allowed in most placed today, including hospitals and clinics. We used to call these animals "Seeing Eye dogs." Animals are available today for all types of assistance. A patient who was blind brought her dog into the clinic when she came for an OB-GYN checkup. Everything went fine until we got ready to do the pelvic exam. As the attending got closer to the patient's pelvis, the dog got closer to the physician. When the speculum got close to the vagina, the dog growled. Finally, the attending told the patient she would have to call him down or hold him in order to perform her pap smear. She did.

The Fate of Most Pagers regarding Males

Most pagers used by male physicians and residents have a short life. There are no old pagers, only new ones. So what happens to pagers regarding males? The urinal in men's restrooms. Men pull down their scrubs in the front to urinate because scrubs do not have zippers. The pager clipped on the waistband slides down to the front of the scrubs and falls off into the urinal. Then, of course, they are no good because they no longer work—and worse, they smell like urine.

So what does one tell the secretary in the medical education office (like she really doesn't know)? It fell into the urinal. One Birmingham hospital gave an award to the resident who lost the most pagers in a urinal. It was not a coveted award.

My First Breech Delivery

In the old days, our program director took clinic and indigent patients who were vertex and turned them by external version to breech. Now a physician would lose his license for doing such and probably be hanged in the town square. The program director felt that knowing how to manage breech deliveries was imperative because eventually one would need to know how. Being skilled with Piper forceps was essential.

My number eventually came up, and it was a typical scenario. An unattached patient presented to labor and delivery about to deliver a breech presentation. There was no time to do a cesarean section or call an attending or chief resident. My luck improved when the charge nurse with four decades' experience asked me how many I had done.

I replied with, "One, counting this one."

She laughed and said not to worry about it because she had done hundreds. I was nervous; she was not.

We took the patient to the delivery room. Before I could worry about it, the patient blew out a term male infant and it was over. Thank goodness!

VI

PRACTICING EMERGENCY MEDICINE IN CARROLLTON, ALABAMA

One of my best educational experiences during residency was working at Pickens County Medical Center in Carrollton, Alabama. I learned a lot and got to do a lot. Most of what I learned, I learned on the spot because it was immediately necessary and no one else was around to help me. Many things I did for the first time without assistance while reading from a book or talking to someone on the telephone. The hospital was in a rural surrounding with a lake behind it and a rolling meadow in the front. Any type of problem could present and usually did. I worked every Tuesday night and two weekends a month from six p.m. on Friday night to five a.m. Monday morning. Then I had to go to my "real job," which was my residency.

Cow at the Emergency Room Door in Pickens County

One day I looked out the door to the emergency department and there stood a cow, just standing there looking in. It stayed there for a while and then wandered off. Maybe it was seeing how busy we were in the ER. I guess she did not have the co-pay. I asked about it and someone said it had gotten out of her fence and regularly came to the emergency department.

Girl with Hole in Her Cheek

One Saturday night, a young woman in her twenties presented to the emergency department complaining of a human bite. Her face was covered by a bloody towel. She stated that she was in a fight with another woman over a man. While they were fighting, the other woman bit her in the face. I removed the towel to find a huge hole in her face. With her mouth closed, you could easily see her teeth and tongue. The hole measured about six centimeters in diameter. A lot of tissue was missing. I told her she needed to see a plastic surgeon to have it repaired, otherwise it was going to heal poorly and she would be disfigured. She asked if I could fix it and I replied I could but it would not look good. She refused to be transferred to a plastic surgeon, so I repaired it. It looked awful and was puckered. She thanked me and left. It looked like she had tetanus.

Vital Signs on Me

I worked in the emergency department at Pickens County Medical Center for a number of years. There was no call room, so the physician on call slept in a regular patient room. On a particularly slow night I went to bed about ten p.m. Shortly after eleven, a nurse came into my room and asked if I needed anything. I said no. I thought, *How nice, they are checking on me.*

Then the nurse said, "I need to get your vital signs."

I asked why.

She said, "Vital signs are taken on everyone."

So I let her take my vital signs. Four hours later, she came in and we went through the whole process again. I finally told her I was the covering physician just sleeping in that room. She said okay.

Postmenopausal Bleeding Patient in the Emergency Department

In the old days, residents took call for a whole weekend—from Friday at seven a.m. until Monday at five p.m. It was grueling. It could be manageable, in which a physician might get some sleep, or a disaster, in which one got no sleep at all. An upper-level resident could have an intern, or a chief may have a second-year or junior resident. Even an acting intern could be helpful.

This particular weekend was a long moonlighting weekend complicated by no sleep at an outlying hospital. Friday and Saturday were busy. Sunday was steady and depressing, on top of my being tired. Sunday night was tricky because not only did you need to get sleep to work the next morning at seven a.m., you had to get up and leave by five to get to the main residency hospital, usually to do surgery.

About ten p.m., the odds of some sleep were promising so I went to bed in the call room. I was exhausted. At one thirty in the morning an elderly lady came to the emergency room with back pain. She did not have a fall or trauma but her chronic pain woke her up. I asked her how long the pain had been going on and she said seventeen years. I asked her what was different tonight (now this morning), and she said she could not stand it any longer. I did a quick exam, X-rayed her spine (which looked okay), and sent her home with some pain medication. Then it was back to bed at two a.m.

At two thirty the emergency department called again, and I was obviously in a deep sleep. The nurse said they had a sixty-five-year-old woman with postmenopausal bleeding. I told the nurse to let her push for an hour, check her cervix, and call me back in an hour. The nurse hesitantly said okay.

In ten minutes the phone rang again, and the nurse asked, "Are you sure that is what you want to do?"

I said, "No. Sorry. I will be right down to see her."

Patient Gets Injection in Parking Lot of Hospital

The state mental hospital called the emergency department and asked if the doctor on call would give an out-of-control psychiatric patient an injection of Thorazine. He could then be better restrained by the men holding him down in the back of a pickup truck and be transported to the mental hospital. This seemed manageable. As the physician looked at the main entrance of the hospital, he saw a pickup truck full of men in the flatbed turn into the hospital driveway. The truck was rocking from side to side. He opened the door, and all he could hear was someone hollering. The pickup drove to the emergency department door. Six stout men were trying to hold the out-of-control psychiatric patient in the bed of the pickup.

Unfortunately, the patient was flinging the six men around in the truck. One of the men asked, "Where do you want us to put him?"

The doctor said, "He will tear up the emergency department. You cannot bring him inside. Just take off his pants here in the parking lot and we will give him a shot here. There are not many people around."

They pulled off his pants in the back of the pickup and gave him the Thorazine injection. The doctor told the men to hurry to the mental hospital. They left as they had arrived, rocking from side to side. For several years after, patients who needed an injection would all ask the same thing, "Can I have my shot in the emergency room, or do I have to pull off my pants and get the shot naked in the parking lot?"

Tick on Tally

When I arrived for a moonlighting shift at a rural hospital one Tuesday night, a general surgeon was completing a chart note. I asked if I needed to see the patient and the response was no. The general surgeon explained that a man showed up with the complaint of something on his penis. The surgeon who was working a shift in the emergency department assumed the man had a wart on his penis. He examined the man to find he had a tick on the head of his penis. The tick was removed. The diagnosis area in the chart read: "Tick on tally."

OB-GYN Has to Drive Ambulance

Moonlighting in a rural hospital often meant transfer of patients to a higher level of care. Ambulance trips were common, and occasionally it was necessary for the emergency department physician to accompany the patient to the tertiary-care hospital forty-five miles away. A husband-and-wife team owned and operated one of the county's two ambulance services. I had been on a lot of trips with them. Neither had great health, but they were dedicated and worked very hard. On one trip, the husband, who was usually the driver, got sick and asked me to drive the ambulance. Having been an EMT, I was glad to drive; it was like the old days.

VII

PRACTICING OBSTETRICS
AND GYNECOLOGY
IN BIRMINGHAM

Early in my career, I practiced at two hospitals in Birmingham, Alabama. One of these was where I had completed my residency; the other was across town. Private practice was an eye-opening experience, especially for a chief resident who thought he knew everything. Fortunately, I continued to learn. Most of all, I learned I did not know everything. All in all, it was enjoyable. It was as much work as residency.

Patient Wants to Marry Dog

The practice of medicine allows physicians to know much about their patients—sometimes more than the physician would wish. I had a pleasant sixty-year-old female patient I had cared for for at least fifteen years. She spent much of her life in a mental hospital, followed by outpatient care in which she lived in a group home. Eventually, she moved into her own home and supported herself on disability assistance.

During one office visit, she announced she was engaged to be married. I congratulated her and inquired about her prospective husband.

She said, "He's black."

I said, "I'm open about biracial marriages." I then asked, "What's his name?"

She replied, "Prince."

I said, "What's his full name?"
She replied, "Prince is his only name."
I thought that was strange. I asked, "What does he look like?"
She said, "He weighs about seventy pounds."
I asked, "Is he healthy?"
She said, "He is."
I replied, "But that's not a good weight for a man."
She said, "He's not a man. He's a dog."
I asked, "Why do you want to do that?"
She said he was protective of her and was never demanding.
I said, "In Alabama, people cannot marry animals."
She continued living a common-law marriage with the dog.

"My Daddy Has a Tail"

By the time most children are in elementary school, they have seen their parents naked. Most notice a difference between their fathers and mothers, whether they acknowledge it or not. Sex education starts early today, and most children know there is a difference between boys and girls.

Early in my career, I had a patient who had four girls. I had delivered three of the girls. None had ever seen their father, or any other man, without clothes.

One of the little girls had walked into the bathroom while her father was urinating. She was horrified and ran out to her mother. She said, "Mommy, my daddy has a tail, and that's nothing—he can tee-tee out of it!"

Natalie Looks up Women's Dresses

As a little girl, Natalie, my youngest daughter, developed the bad habit of trying to look up women's dresses. I regularly disciplined her and even spanked her. I then noticed that it only happened with pregnant women. When Natalie looked up the dress of one of my partners' wives and said, "I want to see the baby," I explained to her that the baby was under the skin, not under the dress. She quit looking.

OB-GYN Patient Asks for a Prostate Examination

Early in my career, I was glad to see any patient who came along as I was building my practice. One Wednesday afternoon, I saw a new patient for a yearly, well-woman checkup. She politely introduced herself and said she was there for a checkup, pap smear, breast exam, and a prescription for her hormones. Pretty straightforward, I thought. The physical examination went well. She had breast implants, but so do many other women. The pelvic examination revealed a lot of scarring. It looked as if she had received radiation therapy to the pelvis. The urethra seemed higher than normal, but maybe that was normal.

I asked the patient if she still had a uterus, and she said no. (This was technically correct because she had never had a uterus.) As I expected, the vagina ended blindly, so I did a pap smear, as was the norm then. Being a good practitioner, I also did a rectal examination, and that is when it got complicated. The patient asked if she could get her prostate checked and that she also needed a prostate specific antigen (PSA) test to screen for prostate cancer. The prostate felt small, but it had been since my internship that I had felt a prostate.

I helped her sit up and said I was missing data in the patient history. So she explained that she'd had a sex change operation twenty years ago. I ordered a mammogram, wrote a prescription for hormones, and told her to expect a letter with the results of her tests in a few weeks. She said, "Thanks. I'll see you next year."

"My Husband Is Very Sick Because He Passes Square Sperm"

In the 1990s, the use of stapling devices to close the uterus at cesarean section became popular. The device consisted of a stapling system inserted in the uterus that was unlocked to deliver the baby and locked back after the baby was delivered. Unfortunately, many women would periodically pass these staples, which looked like square plastic staples, as the uterus healed.

One of our patients was delivered by repeat section and the uterus was opened and closed with the stapling device. The woman did well and went home. Several months later, I saw her in the grocery store and inquired about her baby and husband. She said she and her baby were fine but her husband was very sick. I asked her what was wrong with him. She said she did not know exactly but that he was passing square sperm after intercourse. I told her about the staples, but I am not certain she ever believed me.

Patient Says She Needs to Get Her Cat Checked

Chief residents at their residency graduation think they know everything there is to know about medicine. Most would tackle a tiger if given the opportunity. Many surgery and OB-GYN residents would operate on anything. Nevertheless, the real world awaits them as they enter the practice of medicine. Private practice was an eye-opening experience. There was much I knew nothing about. I suppose that is where the term "lifelong learning" came from.

Older women often refer to their vagina as their "cat" or their "pocketbook," terms I was unfamiliar with. I was happy to see new patients. When you start your practice, everyone is new. A new patient presented with the complaint of, "I need to get my cat checked." My response was that I was not a veterinarian but knew several I could recommend to her. She repeated that she needed to get her cat checked. She said, "You know—my cat." Then my nurse came in and started laughing. She explained that the patient meant her vagina.

"This is a Female Dog—Aren't You a Gynecologist?"

My girls had indoor cats; my son wanted an outside dog. My wife and I finally gave in, and we went to the humane society to find a dog. My son wanted a dog large enough to play with outside. We looked at every animal there. Finally we found him: "Oak Tree." We signed the papers and headed home. Oak Tree was a large dog mix and grew very quickly to more than one hundred pounds. When it was time for shots and a checkup, we headed to a veterinary clinic near our home. One of the veterinarians and his wife were in our Sunday school class. We explained to him that we had gotten this male dog at the humane society and he was our son's new pet.

The vet examined the dog, and when he was finished, said, "Dan, aren't you a gynecologist?"

I said, "Yes, why?"

He said, "This is a female dog!"

Patient Goes Home with Vaginal Speculum Still in the Vagina

The practice of medicine is full of unexpected emergencies, night and day. OB-GYNs are interrupted more than most specialties. Two of us practiced OB-GYN at Norwood Clinic in Birmingham, and the departmental chair practiced gynecology only. The two of us practicing OB-GYN occasionally needed the chair's help in unusual cases, such as cesarean hysterectomies.

One afternoon, the two of us struggled with massive bleeding in a patient and really needed the boss's help. The circulating nurse paged the chair stat to the operating room, and he immediately stopped what he was doing and came. He was in the middle of doing a yearly well-woman visit with a metal Graves speculum in the patient's vagina.

He helped us for several hours and told the office to reschedule his patients. The woman he was examining went home. The next day, the patient called and asked if she could come by and have the metal speculum removed; it was open and still in her vagina.

The receptionist said, "Of course; come in right now."

Overdose on Iron Tablets

Susan was a longtime obstetric patient whom I had cared for for years. I was called to the emergency department for one of my patients, who had overdosed. The patient was Susan. She had a nasogastric tube, and her stomach was pumped out, followed by charcoal administration. The emergency department physician said that Susan was doing okay.

I asked Susan what happened. She replied that her boyfriend had broken up with her and she decided to commit suicide. I asked her what she took, and she said iron tablets. I asked her how many, and she replied the entire bottle. I asked her why she took iron, and she said that was all she had at home.

But iron? She asked what she could expect. I told her her stools would be black and like concrete for about two months, and the security alarm would go off at the airport if she flew anywhere. I also told her it would not be necessary to take iron for a while.

Patient Left in Waiting Room

I was on call at the hospital as an attending physician, and the evening was going well. I had great residents with me that night, and I hoped for a good night. A private patient belonging to one of my partners arrived in labor. Her chart lacked some laboratory tests, so I decided to walk to my office in the nearby professional building to try to find them. I went in through the waiting room and noticed an elderly lady sitting in the corner reading a magazine. She saw me and asked if she was going to be seen soon because she had been there a long time. It was 8:30 p.m. She said that she was supposed to see my senior partner for a well-woman checkup. I knew her physician had already gone home. The staff had also left, and only the cleaning staff was still there. I suspect she had been sitting behind a post and no one realized she was still there. I told her everyone had gone home. I apologized to her and helped her get to her car. She acted like she understood and returned the next morning for her visit.

Orthodontist Gives New Patient a Platter of Milk

During medical school, a fellow student from Tuscaloosa was in dental school. While I studied pathology during residency training, he studied orthodontics and eventually set up a practice in Birmingham. Needing braces, I became his very first patient. Several months into treatment, I went for the usual adjustment. We had the usual conversations, including how expensive it was to set up a dental or orthodontic practice. While adjusting the wires and tightening the bands, the receptionist interrupted us to say a woman was at the front desk wanting braces for her dog. My orthodontist friend told her that the practice did not provide care for animals. The receptionist left but reappeared, saying the woman really wanted to talk to him. Again he said to tell her they did not care for animals.

On the third trip, the receptionist said the woman at the desk was a prominent physician from the University of Alabama in Birmingham Medical Center. She had a show dog with one tooth that needed straightening. She had $5,000 in cash in her purse for a down payment and could bring as much as needed next week. My friend looked around for a minute and then called to the dental assistant, "Mary Jane, please get a platter of milk for one of our new patients!"

Daniel Dials "0" for Emergency Help

Growing up, children learn how to use the telephone. My oldest daughter had friends who called her at home. My son was disturbed that he had no one to talk to or who called him. My daughter had made the observation that even if you do not have anyone to call, if you dial 0, someone will answer whom you can talk to.

During supper that evening, the phone rang and I answered it because I was on call. The voice at the other end identified herself as the operator supervisor at Bellsouth. She said, "Do you need emergency help at your house?"

I quickly said no. She said someone had been calling the operators all afternoon and saying, "Help!" I told her I would make sure it stopped, which I did.

Daniel said he had no one to talk to on the telephone, so he just picked up the phone and dialed 0. I explained to him that was for emergencies only, and I would spank him if he called again.

During Christmas, dads from different streets in our neighborhood would dress like Santa Claus and visit neighborhood children. Before coming, the "Santa" for your street would call parents and ask for information that made him seem real. My older children had fun with it but were old enough to be skeptical. "Santa" showed up and talked to our children on the couch in the living room. My children asked him if he was the real Santa.

"Santa" turned to my son and said, "Daniel, have you been calling the operator anymore and saying 'help'?"

Daniel was stunned. When "Santa" left, Daniel said he was the real Santa because he knew about the emergency phone calls.

Natalie Tells Her Friends I Am an Anesthesiologist

My daughter told me that at school one day, everyone shared with the class what their parents did for a living. She told them that I was a physician. Of course, the teacher asked what kind of doctor. With some hesitation, she told her class that I was an anesthesiologist. Sometime later, Natalie told me what she had done. I asked her why she had told her class I was an anesthesiologist.

My fourteen-year-old daughter said, "Do you think I am going to tell them my father is a gynecologist? You do pap smears and pelvic exams." I took Natalie outside to look at the new Ford Explorer I had just bought her. I told her pap smears had paid for the new truck.

She said, "I see what you mean."

Daniel Makes Money for the Medical Missionaries

In the summertime, many children go to camp for one to two weeks. My son went to a camp associated with our church. It was very nice and well chaperoned, and we were comfortable with him being there. Groups of four boys stayed in cabins, and there was one adult counselor for every four cabins. The counselor would periodically check on the boys. Even though it was church camp, my son's group decided to play poker and bet with the small amount of money they had with them. In the middle of one hand, the counselor walked in. It was obvious what was going on as money and cards were all over the floor. The counselor asked what they were doing. My son, without hesitating, told the counselor they were making money for the medical missionaries. They were all punished, but the counselor said it was all he could do not to laugh about Daniel's quick thinking.

Standing Appointment with the Paramedics

As an OB-GYN, I am called out a lot at night, so we had a security system installed. The blue button called the local police. The red button called the fire department. As the appropriate button was pushed, that agency came to our home as an emergency. Boys love fire trucks. My son learned that pushing the red button made several fire trucks arrive at our home with red lights and sirens on. It became so common that when the Vestavia Fire Department received an alarm to our home, the word at the fire department was, "We need to go to Dan Avery's house!"

Maintenance Man in Bed with Patient

Baptist Medical Center Princeton was synonymous with "great care." Although the hospital was in a terrible section of town, it had survived over the years because of its great care. Obstetrics was no exception, as many pregnant women came to deliver at Princeton. My obstetric practice was large, and I enjoyed every minute of it. We prided ourselves in taking care of many of those who worked at Princeton, as well as their families. It was a friendly atmosphere where almost everyone knew one another.

A very quiet young woman came to see me. Her pregnancy had been uneventful and the delivery went well. Her husband was away when she delivered, so I had not had the opportunity to meet him. The first postpartum morning on rounds, I went in her room to find one of the maintenance men in full Baptist Princeton clothing in bed with her. I roused him up and told him to get out of this patient's bed, that if he got caught, he would be fired! I said, "John, what in the world are doing in this patient's bed?"

The patient then woke and said, "Dr. Avery, this is my husband."

I felt like a fool!

Jesus in the Cafeteria Line at the Hospital

On Sundays, families of attending physicians, residents, and medical students could eat in the cafeteria. I was on call, and my wife and children came to the Baptist Medical Center Princeton for lunch. They had just come from Sunday school and church. My son's lesson had been on Jesus and the little children, and they had seen a picture of Jesus with children playing around him.

We all went through the cafeteria line and sat down to eat. Daniel said, "Dad, Jesus is in the cafeteria line." I asked him where, and he pointed out one of the urologists, who had on scrubs and a long white coat. He had long hair and resembled the picture of Jesus in Sunday school. I told Daniel that was Dr. Bill and he was a urologist. After eating his lunch, Daniel asked if Dr. Bill could play Jesus in the upcoming Christmas play at their school. I told Daniel I would ask him.

Handicapped Patient Slides off Exam Table

One of my first patients after entering private practice was handicapped from a congenital malformation of her hips. She could barely walk yet did not consider herself handicapped. She conceived and presented to my office for obstetric care. Her hip abnormality would not allow her to slide on the examination table, so I had to slip my hands under her hips and pull her down into lithotomy position. We did not discuss this because I just routinely did this at each visit. As the pregnancy advanced and she gained weight, it got harder, but we continued the same procedure with each visit.

The patient eventually delivered by cesarean section because she had a tiny pelvis. She did well, went home, and had a normal postpartum course. She returned for her postpartum checkup, and we went through the usual maneuvers. I did not appreciate that she had lost all her pregnancy weight. When I gave her hips the usual hard tug, she sailed right off the end of the examination table and reflexively wrapped her legs around my head, knocking my glasses off. Her perineum was right on my nose. I grabbed her buttocks in my hands, but they ended up in my lap. I was speechless, and to make it worse, I could not see because my glasses had been knocked off. I lifted her hips back onto the examination table. I asked my nurse for help, but she was laughing so hard she could not help me.

The first thing the patient said was, "I probably can sue you."

I said, "Yes, probably so."

She was uninjured. My prayer was that she would not tell anyone what had happened. I threatened my nurse to keep quiet. Everywhere I went in the hospital, people looked at me and laughed, so I knew the patient had told everyone she knew. Twenty years later and three states away, she called me for a letter of recommendation. By then I could laugh about it.

Napkins—Twenty-Five Cents

Children's activities are abundant today, ranging from prekindergarten through high school. Parents are busy getting children where they need to go.

One Saturday, I carried boys from my son's football team to an out-of-town game. I also helped keep them in line. There were no dressing rooms for boys at the school, so they had to dress in the girls' physical education dressing room.

After the game, we loaded up and headed home. Brown, who was in my son's class, said, "Dr. Avery, do you know what was in the girls' dressing room?"

I said, "No, what?"

Brown said, "Napkins! Why would you have napkins in the girls' dressing room? We have them in our cafeteria, but I've never heard of them in a dressing room! And you know what? They cost twenty-five cents here. Dr. Avery, napkins at our school are free in the cafeteria."

I said, "Brown, better talk to your mother when you get home."

Mother Hands Newborn and Placenta to Hospital Guard

One of our clinic patients called labor and delivery to say she was having regular contractions every five minutes. We told her to come to the hospital because it was her fifth baby and she lived about forty-five minutes away. She'd had very quick labors and deliveries.

She was one mile from the hospital when she delivered a term male infant and placenta in the backseat of their car. She put the baby to her breast to make the uterus contract. The placenta was still attached by the umbilical cord to the baby.

The couple drove into the emergency department entrance portico, and she rolled down the window and handed the newborn baby with placenta and cord attached to the guard. She said she was fine and that they would come back and pick up the baby. They drove off, and the guard was so stunned he did not get the tag number of the car. There was blood all over the guard, as the placenta had rubbed all over his Carraway Hospital blue blazer. There he stood holding a naked newborn baby in his arms without a blanket or anything else with which to warm the baby.

The emergency department called the nursery to come get the baby. There was no name or identification whatsoever. The nursery figured this would be an abandoned baby, who would need to go to the department of human resources.

The baby did well. Three days later, the parents showed up at the nursery door and announced they had dropped off their baby three days earlier and wondered if he was ready to go home. It was not that simple.

Patient Requests Ultrasound Report ASAP

One of the great challenges in medicine is getting laboratory results back to the patient quickly. An obstetric patient named Cassandra asked me, after her ultrasound, to get her results to her as soon as possible. I replied I would.

About three days later, she called me at home around one thirty in the morning for the results. I certainly did not have her results at home. As a matter of fact, I had not seen them. She asked if I was asleep, and I told her I was, but that did not seem to matter. She made me promise that as soon as I saw her report, I would call her with the results. I agreed and tried to go back to sleep.

About an hour later, I was called by a nurse in labor and delivery to tell me I had a patient in labor. By now I had forgotten about the earlier call. I got dressed and went to the hospital. The patient was in labor, so I went to dictate her history and physical. Part of her chart was missing, so I had to go to my office adjoining the hospital to get the full chart. As I went to lock up my office, I saw Cassandra's ultrasound report lying on my desk. I picked up the telephone and called Cassandra. She answered the phone, and I told her I had her ultrasound report for her. She told me she'd been asleep and I had woken her. I told her she had made me promise to call her the minute I saw her report. She replied she did not want to be woken.

Circumcision Is Performed and Head of Penis Falls Off

For centuries, obstetricians have circumcised male newborns, so every OB-GYN and family medicine resident on the obstetric service learned to do "circs."

One morning, I was watching a resident perform a circumcision. Neither I nor the resident knew that different size Gomco clamps had been mixed together. We had a 1.3 clamp and a 1.1 bell. The circumcision went fine.

After removing the clamp, the resident gently removed the bell as appropriate. Blood filled the bell and covered the head of the penis. The resident gently touched the head of the penis and the entire head fell off and rolled across the countertop onto the floor. We were stunned. I saw my life pass in front of me. My career would be over.

Then we looked at the baby's penis. The real head was down under this clot. What had rolled onto the floor was a formed clot in the shape of the head of the penis.

My Son Learns about Sex in Sunday School

One Sunday morning, I went to church in my jeep because I was on call. My family went in my wife's car. You know how it is—if we had gone together, I would have been called out. Since we were in separate vehicles, I did not receive any pages. My son asked if he could ride home with me. He was eight years old. We loaded up and headed home.

Before we could get out of the parking lot, Daniel said, "Dad, you're not going to believe what Michael told me in Sunday school."

I said, "What?"

Michael told him if a boy puts his penis in a girl's vagina, she could get pregnant. He said, "Dad, tell me that is not true."

I said, "Daniel, it is pretty much the truth."

Stunned he said, "Dad, you can count on me; I will never do anything like that."

I said, "Great, let's get that in writing when we get home and get it notarized! You might change your mind."

"Doctor, I Have Had an Autopsy Performed on Me"

I saw a new patient in the office for a checkup. I went through all the components of a history and physical. When I got to previous surgeries, she listed the following: craniotomy, cervical fusion, thyroidectomy, cardiac bypass surgery, angiogram, mitral valve replacement, carotid endarterectomy, mastectomy, breast biopsy, breast reduction, laparoscopic cholecystectomy, partial gastrectomy, splenectomy, appendectomy, bilateral tubal ligation, dilatation and curettage, myomectomy, ovarian cystectomy, total vaginal hysterectomy, bilateral salpingo, oophorectomy, anterior and posterior colporrhaphy, hemorrhoidectomy, colonoscopy, arthroscopy, bilateral knee replacement, open reduction internal fixation of tibia, cataract extraction, face lift, myringotomies, lung biopsy, and chest tube.

She said, "You know, when you think about it, I have pretty much had an autopsy done on me because I have had so many surgeries done! There could not be much left."

Oncology Service Complains about Brahms's "Lullaby"

Women typically make the health-care decisions for their families. Most hospitals invest heavily in marketing obstetric and gynecologic services. If a woman is happy with her obstetric care, she usually will return with subsequent pregnancies. She will take her children to that hospital. She will take her husband for a vasectomy. Hospitals therefore want the labor and delivery service to be wonderful. Most hospitals make a big "to-do" over a delivery, and many today play Brahms's "Lullaby" after a delivery so the whole hospital can celebrate the delivery.

A hospital where I practiced a long time traditionally played Brahms's "Lullaby" after a delivery. But after a few years, the oncology service wanted equal time. They demanded that if the obstetrics service played "Lullaby" after a delivery, they wanted a hymn played after a death. They wanted "When We All Get to Heaven" played. The hospital administration responded by not playing either.

Patient Is Pronounced Dead by Attending but Is Later Alive

Today, most people expire at the hospital. A patient on the gastrointestinal service was at death's door, and the family had been called to his bedside. The patient's nurse had called the attending because she could no longer detect any vital signs. The attending told the nurse to bring the family into the conference room. His plan was to talk to them after he pronounced the patient dead. He saw the patient and determined the time of death. As he talked to the family and explained that the patient, whose death was not unexpected, had died, the nurse appeared in the door of the conference room motioning for the attending. Understanding that time with the family was more important than what the nurse may have wanted, he continued talking with the family. Even though they had expected the worst, the family members were crying and praying to God to restore life to their loved one.

At the conclusion of the meeting with the patient's family, the physician left the room, only to find the nurse waiting for him. She said the patient was moving around and was not dead. The physician quickly went to the patient's room to confirm the same. What was he going to do? He had just spent thirty minutes with the family explaining why the patient had died.

He hurried back to the conference room and announced, "Your prayers have been answered; your father is alive now!"

Elderly Patient "Karate Chops" Paramedics

A sixty-year-old lady I had taken care of for years was discharged from the state mental hospital into a group home. She progressed to independent living in a home by herself. For some reason, she decided to take karate lessons, as she was in pretty good physical health. I did not think the lessons would last, but after a few years she had worked up to a black belt, believe it or not.

One day she called me and said she was having chest pain. I told her to call an ambulance, as she lived alone, and reluctantly, she did so. The paramedics responded quickly to her home, with red lights and siren on, and ran to her front door, not knowing what to expect. Now, my patient was a little different, I guess from living in a state mental hospital for years. The paramedics thought she was drunk by her voice and actions and accused her accordingly. She became angry and performed a few karate chops on both of the paramedics, significantly injuring one of them. The paramedics ran from her, got in the ambulance, and left without her.

She called me back saying her pain was worse and told me about what had happened. I called the ambulance company and they refused to go back to her home—not only this time but forever. The company said that they had posted a list in the dispatcher's office of patients who had harmed them. She was now on the list. I called a Yellow Cab, who picked her up and took her to the hospital.

Award at Baptist Hospital for Destroying Telephones

Hospitals give all kinds of awards to physicians, some to reward good behavior and some to entice better behavior. The Baptist Hospital gave an award for the physician who had destroyed more telephones the previous year than any other physician. The award actually made fun of a single physician who destroyed the most telephones. The same physician received the award every year. He had a miserable temper and in today's world would be labeled a disruptive physician. As the story goes, he founded the cardiology department, brought in three cardiovascular surgeons, got a certificate of need for cardiovascular bypass surgery, and was instrumental in a new heart transplant program. He was one of the top admitters to the hospital. The administration's approach was to do nothing; after all, it was easy to replace telephones.

Children Watch OB-GYN Educational Videos

Marketing companies often send materials for physicians to view, hoping they will purchase some of them. I had received three educational videos: a natural birth with anesthesia, a forceps delivery under epidural anesthesia, and a repeat cesarean section. I took them home to look at before I went to bed, and I put them on my side of the bed. My wife had been to the video store and rented three movies for the children. She put her three movies on her side of the bed.

At the conclusion of dinner, she announced to our three children that she had movies for them to watch. They disappeared to their rooms. My wife and I finished dinner and cleaned up the kitchen. I went to the bedroom, and my videos were missing. I noticed the children's videos were still on her side of the bed. I knew where my videos were.

I walked into the playroom to see my children's eyes as big as saucers. They were watching the deliveries, and they were horrified. Daniel asked how the vagina stretches that much for a head to come out. That night we started talking about sex. I had not planned to, but it was time. My children were full of questions. First and foremost was how mothers get pregnant.

Worms in the Christmas Cookies

It was Christmastime, and four of us who had trained together at Carraway Methodist Medical Center started a new practice as OB-GYNs at Baptist Princeton and Bessemer Carraway Medical Centers. We were the new kids on the block. Marketing seemed important to get our new practice rolling. We wanted to be a household name in the local medical profession. It seemed prudent to do something for prospective referring physicians at both of these hospitals. But what?

My three children came home from school and announced their school was selling Christmas cookies to raise money for some worthy project. They each had to sell a certain quota of tins of cookies. I had a great idea: I could kill not two but three birds with one stone. Our practice would buy three hundred tins of cookies. The children would more than meet their quotas. We would give those cookies to the referring physicians. Best of all, I could get a tax break by taking the cost of the cookies as a business expense on my income tax.

The cookies came in a round tin with Christmas decorations. We added a bow and a card expressing Christmas wishes from all of us. We all participated in delivering the tins. The interesting thing was that as the days went by and we got closer to Christmas, no physician said a word about the cookies, not one. It was kind of frustrating. We wondered if we had insulted someone. Then the answer came.

One of the internists at Bessemer Carraway saw me in the hall at the hospital. He said, "You know those cookies that you gave me were full of worms!"

I was speechless and really did not know how to respond other than saying I was so sorry and to explain where we had gotten the cookies. We sent Christmas cards the next year.

Fire at Princeton OB-GYN PC

Every morning was busy in the clinic. One of my partners, Dr. Denson, commented that he had smelled smoke all morning at his end of the office. He came and got me, and sure enough, there was a smoky smell. We looked everywhere. We thought it worthwhile to look for a fire before calling the fire department and evacuating the building.

Dr. Denson and I looked outside the back door of our building and saw the culprit. It was summertime, and there was dried sawdust around the shrubbery. A lit cigarette had been thrown into the sawdust and set it on fire. The fire was not that big. We thought we would try our hand at extinguishing it before calling Birmingham Fire and Rescue.

We went back into our building and opened the fire extinguishing closet, and there was a fire extinguisher and a fire hose attached to a water line. Of course we chose the fire hose. It was every man and boy's dream—shoot water from a fire hose. We pulled the hose out and aimed at the fire outside the building. I turned on the water. There was more pressure in the line than we expected. I could understand why it takes several firemen to hold a fire hose spraying water. We got dirty and wet and had to put on scrubs. The fire was out.

"Don't You Think It's Fair That We See You Naked?"

During a third cesarean section late one evening, I developed substernal chest pain. I was able to complete the procedure and immediately went to the emergency department downstairs, where I was promptly evaluated. Unfortunately, I was given Dilaudid, to which I am allergic.

I remember waking up and hearing a medical student say, "He still does not have a pulse or blood pressure. Why do you think he was jerking his arms and legs like that?"

I was in deep trendelenburg position (in which my feet were highly elevated), and I had a headache. I remember the emergency physician saying they were admitting me to the ICU, and I would have a cardiac catheterization the next day. The charge nurse called my wife to tell her I was being admitted, and she told the nurse she would see me tomorrow, expecting everything to be all right. She also called one of my partners to take call for me.

The next morning my son called me and asked if I would shoot basketball with him when I got home, and I told him I would. He asked me if I did not make it, could he have my watch. I said sure.

The cardiac catheterization was next. I got there and the lab was freezing. All the ladies in the cath lab were patients of mine, and it helped me feel more comfortable. My cardiologist gave me some Versed, and I felt crazy.

The next thing I knew I was basically naked except for a blanket over my upper torso and arms. The technician told me she was going to prep me, and she came at me with what looked like a razor that was a foot wide. I had never seen a razor that big. She started swinging it at my groin, and I yelled, "You are going to cut my little buddy off!" One of the nurses stepped up and said, "Don't you think it's fair that we see you naked? After all, you have seen all of us naked." I had cardiac catheterization performed and my heart was normal.

Patient Wants Epidural but Husband Says "No!"

Most women today labor and deliver with epidural anesthesia. Occasionally, there are women who want to go "natural." Some of these do it for a while, and some do it all the way. A patient came to the labor room in great pain from advanced dilatation and asked for pain relief, but her husband said no! I asked her what she wanted, and she said she would do what he wanted. He explained he was an active-duty marine, and all his contemporaries' wives had had "no anesthesia and went natural" and he wanted his wife to do that also.

She continued to suffer. While he stepped out to use the restroom, the patient asked me if I could get my hands on a large sharp-teethed clamp. I told her that I had a Willet clamp at the desk. It was a large clamp with a row of large sharp teeth at the end used for grasping bone.

She said, "Will you bring it in my room when my husband gets back?"

I said I would and I did.

She said, "Dr. Avery, I am experiencing natural labor and childbirth for my husband. I want him to enjoy it too. Will you put that large, sharp clamp on his scrotum?"

I said, "Sure, pull your pants down."

He was stunned and asked me to step out of the room, and I did. He followed me out about three minutes later. He said, "My wife needs an epidural."

I replied, "Smart man!"

Patient Delivers at Home and Husband Is Distraught

Carolyn called me and said she was in labor. I told her to come in because she lived about an hour from the hospital, down near the river, and had had previous quick labors. Five minutes later, she called back, and I could hear a baby crying in the background.

She said, "Dr. Avery, I had this baby in the bed. It's already here."

I asked where her husband was. She said he was in his boxers running outside around the house because she had scared him to death.

I told her to wrap up the baby and when Leroy settled down, to come to the hospital.

Admitted for a Kidney Stone and Made a DNR

Kidney stones and I are not friends. I had my first stone the last week of residency. It was obstructing, and I was admitted to the hospital my last week of residency. It culminated in a stone-basket procedure with a perforated ureter. I can remember trying to take the written board exam and falling asleep.

Several years later, I had another stone, and being unable to pass it, went to the emergency department and was admitted. The clerk went through the whole deal about power of attorney, whether I wanted to be resuscitated, etc. To my amazement, my wife said she did not want me to be resuscitated. She wanted me to be a "DNR," or "Do Not Resuscitate." I said, "I am just here for a kidney stone and want to be resuscitated. I am not even forty years old." I guess I should have appreciated that my marriage was in trouble but did not know it.

Homeless Fourteen-Year-Old Drives Fire Truck

At a family reunion, a distant relative told me an incredible story about his upbringing. For whatever reason, his mother could not care for him, and he had to leave home. This happened many years ago before welfare, children's services, and the department of human resources. He gathered his belongings and lit out from a fairly respectable neighborhood in Birmingham. He passed by the one volunteer fire station, and the firemen gave him a bed. After that, he actually lived at the fire station but went to school during the day. This was his home, and the firemen were his family. By age fourteen, he was pretty good at putting out fires. So the fire chief gave him a letter, which he carried with him all the time. The letter said that he was authorized to drive the fire truck to fires; he was fourteen. This worked out well because he was the only one at the fire station at night, since it was a volunteer department. The volunteer firemen just met him at the fire, which saved time. He later became a paramedic and has recently retired.

Patient Delivers Baby at Black Market Baby Farm

I was seeing a patient in the emergency department at Carraway Methodist Medical Center. One of the nurses asked me to look at another patient's perineum. She said the internal medicine service was admitting a patient with Rocky Mountain spotted fever. The nurse was supposed to obtain a catheterized urine specimen for urinalysis and culture. She said the patient's perineum had several lacerations. She said it looked exactly like someone who had just given birth. She asked the patient if she had just delivered a baby. The patient said no, she had never been pregnant or even had sex. The nurse was perplexed. She was holding the urine specimen she had obtained, and we did a pregnancy test on it, which was positive. I called the medicine resident and told him what we knew. He then consulted the OB-GYN service.

I went in and introduced myself to the patient. I explained that the nurse was concerned about the lacerations on her bottom. She again said she had not been pregnant and had never had sex. I examined her. It looked exactly like someone who had just given birth. There were perineal lacerations typical of a vaginal delivery. The cervix was floppy and the uterus was about twenty weeks' size. I told her that her pregnancy test was positive, which would stay positive for several weeks after delivering a baby.

More emphatically I asked, "Where is the baby?"

She said, "There is no baby."

I told her I was paging the hospital attorney and security, who in turn would call the police and the FBI. This would play out like a murder because a baby was missing.

She said, "This is what happened. I got pregnant. I was scared to death. I wore loose clothes and hid the pregnancy from my mother, who I lived with. She never figured it out. As I started having occasional contractions, I knew I had to do something. My mother and I could not afford a baby because we could hardly exist as it is. Someone told me about someone you could call and get rid of your baby. I called the number and a man said that he could help me. It would cost me $300. I got the money and called him back. He gave me a place to be in North Birmingham. When he picked me up, he blindfolded me. He told me for his protection, I had to stay blindfolded until we got to our destination. We got to a farm in some rural area. We went in this house, and they took my money. I asked exactly what was going to happen to me. The man, who they called 'the doctor,' would induce me and deliver my baby. They showed me around. I was the only pregnant woman there. There were about seven or eight cribs lined up together in one room. All contained what looked like newborn babies.

"I was put to bed. They gave me medicine in my arm, and I started contracting. I labored without anything for pain. The 'doctor' and a woman delivered my baby and took it away. They gave me medicine to make me stop bleeding. I stayed there for a few hours. Then they blindfolded me again and loaded me up and took me back to where they had picked me up. I got a friend to take me home. My bottom is torn up, and they did not sew me up. I did all right for a while but then started running a fever. When the fever got to 103 degrees, I decided to come to the emergency room."

To make a long story short, the admitting diagnosis was toxic shock syndrome, and she was admitted to the ICU. The FBI and police handled the investigation and found where she had delivered the baby, which was a black market baby farm preying on young pregnant women who did not want to keep their babies.

"I Do Not Know Who the Father Is"

In the 1960s, it was unusual to have a patient say she did not know who the father of the baby was; today it is common. We have traditionally relied on blood group testing of the mother, baby, and possible father to help determine if a male could be the father or at least exclude him as a possibility. DNA testing in recent years has allowed determination of the father of a baby to the odds of one in one million. Patients often want to know by ultrasound the exact day that conception occurs to help them sort out early in the pregnancy who could be the father. One patient wanted me to tell her if she got pregnant Tuesday, Wednesday, or Thursday evening. Of course, ultrasound is not that specific.

One patient told me she did not know who the father was but could narrow it down to three men. Her plan was to see who the baby looked like after delivery. No one was present with her during labor and delivery. After the baby was born, she asked me to take the baby to the obstetrics waiting room. I did exactly that. I went to the waiting room and announced the mother's name. Three gentlemen were sitting together, and all three got up together and came to look at the baby. She selected the father based on who the baby favored, and he became the daddy.

You Can Make a Baby in Three Months

I went to see my grandmother. She said, "You know technology today is incredible."

I asked, "What do you mean?"

She said, "In my day, it took nine months to make a term baby. Today, you can do it in much less time. Your cousin Elizabeth got married three months ago yesterday. Today, they had a seven-pound term baby girl who was healthy. The technology will allow you to have a term baby in three months that normally would have taken nine."

I realized what my grandmother was implying and just laughed. I replied, "I'm glad they are doing fine."

VIII

PRACTICING OBSTETRICS AND GYNECOLOGY IN WINFIELD

My greatest contribution to medicine has been practicing in rural Alabama. I started practicing medicine in Winfield, Alabama, by working in the Carraway Northwest Medical Center emergency department during residency. I worked there part-time in obstetrics and gynecology after residency until moving there permanently after fellowship training.

Elvis Is Alive and Delivers Baby in Winfield

As country obstetricians, our group made every effort to deliver as many of our own patients as possible. Sometimes it meant laboring a patient and then calling her regular doctor just before delivery. Despite all efforts, sometimes that was not possible. My partner had a social event he very much wanted to attend but knew a special patient was probably in labor. The social event was a fund-raiser and included costumes. My partner was dressed like Elvis Presley, and I must say, he looked very much like him.

He arrived at the social function in a limousine. Sure enough, while my partner was at the party, the patient went into active labor. So I called my partner and told him the news. My plan was to labor the patient, and when she was close to delivery, call him to come in and deliver the baby.

The labor went quicker than expected. When she said she felt pressure, I checked her, and the baby's head was right at the perineum.

I told her not to push so I could call her doctor. He sped to the hospital in the limousine to do the delivery.

Here is what people at the hospital saw: a speeding limousine slides in to the entrance of the hospital, and Elvis jumps out and runs into the delivery room. There was no time to change into scrubs, so he delivered the baby in his costume. The baby was fine, the delivery uncomplicated. The door opens and Elvis is holding the newborn. The patient told Elvis to go back to the party. I agreed to clean up, write a delivery note, and sign orders. The public saw Elvis run out of the hospital, get into his limousine, and speed off.

Headlines the next day read: "Elvis Is Alive and Delivers Baby in Winfield!"

Couple Has Sex in Examination Room after Office Visit

A couple came to see me for a thirty-nine-week prenatal visit. The patient had a routine, low-risk pregnancy that had gone well. The nurse saw them first and took vital signs, including weight and a urine dip for glucose and protein. My part of the visit went well. The baby had a good fundal height and good heart tones. I checked the patient's cervix, and it was closed. This was their first baby, and the couple was anxious to deliver. They asked me about how to accelerate cervical ripening and dilatation. We discussed the usual ways: walking, spicy foods, and the like. They asked me about sex, and I told them that many thought that helped. I told them to see me in a week if they had not delivered and left the room.

I saw several other patients and did not notice that the couple never came out of the exam room despite the fact that the room was right by the nurses' station. My nurse came to me when she realized they had never come out. She opened the door and was speechless. The wife was still undressed in the stirrups. The husband was standing at the step on the bottom of the exam table with his pants pulled down. He was holding on to her legs in the stirrups. They were having sex right in the unlocked exam room. My stunned nurse asked them what they were doing. They did not answer, but the husband pulled up his pants and the nurse shut the door.

They both came out smiling and said, "See you next week."

"Bring Your Prescription Pad to the Family Reunion"

When you graduate from residency, everyone wants you to write them a prescription for whatever. They are completely ignorant of the fact that there are rules about whom you can write a prescription for. My turn came when an uncle called the day before a family reunion and asked me to bring my prescription pad to the reunion. I thought it was a strange request. I asked why I needed to do that, and he said that everyone in the family had medications they wanted. I did not take a prescription pad with me the next day to the reunion. The uncle got to me first and was disappointed when I told him I did not bring a prescription pad.

Out of curiosity, I asked him what he needed, and he replied Librium. I asked him how long he had been on the medication, and he said, "Forty-five years." I asked him how many he needed and he replied, "How about a thousand?"

Dumping Patient off Electric Table onto the Floor

In the 1980s and '90s, electric tilting examination tables became popular. Unfortunately, they were very expensive, costing about $10,000 apiece, compared to $600 for a regular stationary exam table. Most could only afford a few of the electric exam tables or maybe just one. The tables were great for procedures, colposcopies, endometrial biopsies, or even for handicapped or paralyzed patients.

The trick to operating the table was understanding the controls. My first patient sat down in the chair, and I hit the controls. The patient's legs went easily into the supine position, but as I hit the other floor pedals, the bed began tilting up, so the patient slid right onto the floor. To make matters worse, she was pregnant! Fortunately, she was unharmed.

Dog in Delivery Room

Obstetrics has changed dramatically during my career. When I was a medical student, husbands were not allowed in the labor room. The husband's place was to sit in the waiting room and smoke cigarettes while his wife was in labor. The mother, upon arrival to the labor room, received 100 mg of Demerol and half an ampule of scopolamine, all through an IV. She would not have recognized her husband anyway. He certainly did not get to go into the delivery room, because the mother was asleep from cyclopropane. The nurse pushed on the fundus, and the physician pulled out the baby with forceps. The nurse carried the newborn baby out to the waiting room for the father to see. He immediately changed from cigarettes to cigars. Four to five days later, the mother woke up, saw her new baby for the first time, and was discharged.

Now, everyone is allowed in the labor and delivery rooms. Sometimes many people are present, including friends, relatives, and even the minister on occasion. One of my patients wanted to have her dog in the delivery room. I asked if she was blind or if it was an assistance dog, but said it was not. I asked her why she wanted the dog in the room for the delivery and she told me he was the family pet and she wanted it to be a good experience for him. I asked, "Who cares? No dog in the delivery room!" You have to draw the line somewhere!

"I Need to Know How to Have Sex"

As a country doctor, I learned to not be surprised by anything. When I thought I had heard everything, there would be an even more astounding story.

One Friday afternoon, a nurse from the operating room called and said she had to be seen because it was an emergency. I knew we were busy and employees were anxious to go home. Nevertheless, I answered that it would be okay for her to come to my office. At 4:55 p.m. I entered her room. She looked calm, although I did not know what to expect. She did not look distressed. I said, "What can I do for you?"

She said, "The rehearsal dinner is tonight, and I am getting married tomorrow. I need to know how to have sex."

I said, "What do you already know?"

She said, "Nothing."

I went out to the nurses' station and told my employees to go on home, that I was going to be a while.

I went back in and asked if she and her fiancée had kissed, and she said yes. We went through the whole process of foreplay, undressing, the hymen, intercourse, and contraception. She did not seem that excited. I commended her on waiting to have sex until she got married. I guess everything worked out okay because she now has two children.

Family Members Stand around Bed with Lit Candles

Late one afternoon, after seeing all my office patients, I made postoperative rounds at the hospital. The last patient I went in to see presented an unusual situation. It was a patient of one of my colleagues, whom I was covering for. I went in, and the room was full of family members. They were lined up around the bed, side by side, on both sides and at the foot, holding lit candles. It was very quiet, so I just backed out of the room and decided to come back later. I thought what I saw probably had something to do with their church or religious preference.

One of the family members followed me out into the hall. I asked her what was going on and she replied that the patient had "gas." I asked what were the candles being used for, and she said they helped with the awful smell of the gas she was passing. I told her my concerns were the ten open flames of the candles and the oxygen on the wall that could explode.

Nurse Faxes Her Breasts to OB-GYN

Donita was an excellent registered nurse in labor and delivery, but she was also a party animal and the social director of the service. If there was a party, she was there. When one of the OB-GYNs commented on the telephone about her breasts, she said she would fax them to him. How do you fax breasts? She went into the computer room, shut the door, pulled up her scrub top and bra, pressed her bare breasts onto the copier screen, and hit the copy and fax button, sending "her breasts" to the OB-GYN in his office. I had never seen this done before, and it caused quite a stir. Rural health can be very exciting from time to time! This is also the nurse who claimed she always had sex on the first date "if he looked okay."

Obstetric Patient Has a Toothache

At two o'clock one morning, a patient called complaining of a toothache. I recognized her name and exchanged pleasantries. I asked her about her tooth pain. I told her it sounded to me like she needed to see her dentist. She replied that she had that day and he had done a root canal. I asked if he had given her anything for pain. She said Percocet. I asked if she had taken any and she said she took two tablets an hour ago. She said she was still hurting. I asked her why she had not called her dentist, and she said that she did not want to wake him up. She figured that since I was an OB-GYN, I was probably up anyway.

Patient Gets Urine Sample for Me

My practice of obstetrics and gynecology in Winfield, Alabama, has been the height of my professional career. An OB-GYN by training, I was also the primary-care provider for more than half my patients. We routinely did four CLIA-waived laboratory tests in my office: dip urinalysis, pregnancy tests, hemoccults, and wet preps.

I saw a patient who was having dysuria (bladder inflammation). I asked her to provide me with a urine sample, which she agreed to do. She was sitting on the exam table in a gown. As I left the room, she jumped down from the table, pulled up her gown, squatted on the floor, and urinated in the middle of the floor. When I returned, there was a puddle of urine in the middle of the floor. I asked her why she did not urinate in a cup. She said I did not tell her to use a cup.

No Speeding Tickets for Doctors, Nurses, and Food Handlers

Over time, I have had the opportunity to care for, deliver, and operate on law enforcement officers, their spouses, and their children. Many I have taken care of for long periods of time. I have been stopped by law enforcement officers on many occasions but have only gotten one ticket over the years. I am usually stopped for speeding, but the one ticket I got was for running a red light in Birmingham.

While his wife was in labor, I discussed this with a state trooper assigned to the small town where I practiced. He laughed and explained why I had only gotten one ticket. He said that law enforcement officers usually do not give tickets to doctors and nurses because they may need treatment from them in an emergency situation at the emergency room. I asked, "What about food handlers?" He said, "They usually do not get tickets either. They might put something in your food."

Husband Tries to Leave Wife with Bad PMS at My Home

Living in a small town was great and quite rewarding. But you have to accept that everyone knows everything about you. They know where you live and where you go. Patients even drop by your home, especially when you are outside working in the yard or cutting grass.

There was one particular patient I was treating who had terribly painful PMS. She was making some progress but still had a long way to go. While cutting grass, I noticed a white Buick turning into my driveway and coming toward my house. I tried to watch out of the corner of my eye. I saw my patient get out of the passenger side, and the husband was in the driver's seat.

I figured it was time to walk over and see what was up.

The husband said, "Doc, she's not much better. Can I just leave her with you and your wife until she gets better?"

She was getting out of the car and had her suitcase with her.

I said, "No, my wife won't let us do that."

Physician Stopped by Winfield Police but Not for Speeding

Despite public opinion, physicians actually get sick from time to time. Doctors and nurses usually treat themselves rather than going to the doctor like the rest of the world. When one treats himself, he has a "fool for a doctor and a fool for a patient," as the saying goes. Nevertheless, I was recovering from the flu and had just started back to work. In a small town, everyone knows everything about you, whether you like it or not. It is more fun when the topic of conversation is not you. People know you have diarrhea if you buy Pepto-Bismol in the Junior Food Mart. They know you are constipated if you buy Correctol. If you are single and buy condoms, they feel compelled to know who the lucky partner is.

I was driving home one day, minding my own business, not speeding or anything. I heard a siren behind me and pulled off the road to let the emergency vehicle pass. Physicians are most often stopped by the police for exceeding the speed limit going to the hospital to attend an emergency.

The police car stopped right behind me, its red and blue lights flashing. *This is unfortunate,* I thought, *because everyone in town will know and my patients passing by will question my competency if I am stopped by the police.* I got my driver's license and registration out and rolled down the window.

The policeman I knew well because he was also a paramedic, and I was his daughter's physician. I courteously asked him what I had been doing wrong. He said, "Nothing, of course!" He said he heard I'd been sick and wanted to know if I was doing better. He saw me in afternoon traffic and wanted to catch up to talk. He figured the best way was to make an emergency run with lights and siren. I thanked him for his concern and eased on home.

"Are You Using Those Posthole Diggers on Me?"

Some of my most memorable experiences in medicine come from outlying clinics. No doubt I have enjoyed taking care of many women for many years. One of my elderly patients always called vaginal speculums "posthole diggers" because she said the speculum resembled that tool. At each yearly visit, she always said, "Are you using those posthole diggers on me?" I always answered, "Yes."

Stopped by the Carbon Hill Police

One Friday afternoon right after lunch, I was driving to Birmingham for the weekend to see my children who lived there. As I drove through Carbon Hill, I heard a siren and looked in my rearview mirror to see a Carbon Hill police car behind me, its red and blue lights flashing. I pulled over. I knew I was not speeding and wondered if I'd been going too slow. I had on hospital scrubs.

The officer came to the driver's window and told me to get out. He pushed me down and placed my hands on the hood. Carbon Hill is about ten miles from where I practiced, and I could see people I knew riding by.

I asked, "What have I done?"

The policeman said nothing.

By now, a second police car pulled up, also with siren and lights flashing. The officer said they had received a report of a blue Chevrolet SUV filled with teenagers throwing out paper onto the highway. I said, "Officer, I'm by myself, I'm fifty years old, I have no paper, and I'm driving a white Ford Explorer."

The two officers went to the patrol car and talked. They came back and said I could go.

Pre-antibiotic Treatment for Postpartum Mastitis

Necessity is the mother of invention. My grandmother told me so much about medicine and childbirth, I wished I had her back to ask more questions. One time, for some reason, she and I got to talking about breast-feeding, which was the norm in her day. She asked me about the treatment of mastitis, and we discussed antibiotics. When she had children, there were no antibiotics. She told me that when she or any other woman got mastitis, they quit nursing on the affected side. They got a newborn puppy and nursed it on the affected breast and nursed her baby on the unaffected breast. This continued until the breast cleared of infection. This treatment was called "getting a puppy."

Woman Catches Trichomoniasis from Cat

I have had the pleasure of working with my wife in my office. In the evenings after dinner, she made many of the calls to patients, answering messages and calling in prescriptions. One pregnant patient was found to have trichomoniasis on a pap smear. She was in the second trimester, and I asked my wife to call her in a prescription of Flagyl after talking to the patient. The patient replied that she had gotten the "trich" from a cat. My nurse then explained that a pregnant woman may catch toxoplasmosis from a cat. Trichomoniasis came from sexual contact, and both she and her significant other needed treatment. The patient said she understood and appreciated having the prescription being called in. Then she asked, "How much Flagyl should I give the cat?"

Postoperative Instructions about Sexual Intercourse

It was postoperative day number three and time to go home after performing a total abdominal hysterectomy. The patient had done well and had no complications. So I went through the usual course of what to do and what not to do. My patient was attentive. Sitting with her was a well-groomed gentleman about her age that I assumed to be her husband, since the patient started asking questions about intercourse. I went through the precautions and how long to wait. I turned the man and told him to be easy the first time or two when he inserted. I also told him to avoid deep thrusting.

The patient then said, "This is Reverend Lee. He is the pastor of my church."

I was speechless.

Laboring Patient Pushes While Eating a Chicken Leg

Despite all good intentions, the wrong diet was delivered to a patient in labor. In fact, she was pushing with her legs in the stirrups. No one else was in the room, so she dug in and started eating. I came into the room to check her and found her pushing while simultaneously eating a chicken leg.

I told her not to eat, and she replied she was starving.

Minister Comes to Visit Me after Surgery

During part of the time I was a country obstetrician, I was single. My wife of many years did not like rural life and chose another path for her future. I was committed to medical care in a rural town in West Alabama. I did some dating here and there. Unfortunately, in a small town, everyone knows your business. Nevertheless, I loved the area, my patients, the care that the physicians gave, my house, my friends, and my life. However, when I needed surgery on my neck for a herniated disk, I wondered how I would survive. My partner was wonderful, doing as much as he could. The nurses in labor and delivery took great care of me as well, bringing meals and checking on me.

One evening, the nurses in labor and delivery prepared dinner for me. It was delivered by a single nurse who was fun-loving. We were great friends, and I'd never dated her. She decided to wrap the meal in a pair of her black thong panties. After a few laughs, she took the panties off the tray of food and left them lying on couch. She then put dinner on my kitchen table and left. We both forgot about the panties.

Later that evening, the pastor of my church came to visit me. I invited him into the living room, and he sat down. The panties were still lying on the couch. He could not help but see them. He never acknowledged it, but he couldn't have missed them. I'm not sure what I expected him say—maybe something like, "My wife has a pair like that," or "Who do those belong to?" or "Did you have company earlier?"

Grandmother First Assists with Stat Cesarean Section

The hospital where I trained was an eight-hundred-bed teaching facility, with every specialty except pediatric cardiovascular surgery. There was always more than enough manpower. This was not the case in rural Alabama hospitals, with bed counts ranging from twenty to one hundred. I had done cesarean sections with nurse anesthetists, nursing students, paramedics, and medical students.

One Friday night I had a unique opportunity. We were busy in labor and delivery and, of course, were short of help. We had several deliveries going on at the same time. I was laboring the daughter of one of the scrub technicians from the operating rooms.

As is often the case in obstetrics, the baby's heart tones dropped to the fifties. Nothing we did helped. So the nurse anesthetist and I ran to the section room, as my nurse was doing another delivery. We got the patient on the table, and I prepped her quickly. I donned a surgical hat, mask, gown, and gloves. The patient already had an epidural. The problem was, I had no help whatsoever.

The baby's grandmother-cum-scrub tech, seeing the situation from the observation window, ran in, gowned, and gloved. She said, "Let's go!"

The baby was out in a minute and did well. The mother closed well. The pediatrician arrived and cared for the baby.

The grandmother pulled off the surgical garb, and leaving the room, said she had hoped to see the delivery, but not that close. I was grateful and thanked her.

Man Does Not Dress after Biopsy of His Penis

The human papillomavirus (HPV) has changed the entire picture of pap smears. I remember one of the GYN oncologists at University Hospital discovering the virus, visualizing clear areas in the cytoplasm thought to be HPV. A large amount of work was done learning how to manage HPV infections and abnormal pap smears. It soon became apparent that men were subjected to this as well. While we colposcoped and biopsied women's cervices, we also needed to examine men.

A urologist wrapped the penis of a man thought to have HPV with cloths soaked with acetic acid (such as the method for colposcopy, where we then look for lesions with the colposcope). Then came the kicker: should men have their penises biopsied? For a short period, colposcopy of the penis went okay, but biopsy of the penis did not. In fact, most men did not get dressed after a biopsy because it was so painful. They immediately got up, grabbed their clothes, and ran out, mostly naked. None returned for the pathology report. Today, urologists have stopped randomly biopsying the penis.

Guaranteed Method of Getting Family Members to Give Blood

"Transfusion medicine" (or transfusiology, the branch of medicine concerned with the transfusion of blood and blood components) has not always had the sophistication it has today. Blood banking in the 1950s and 1960s had significant limitations, and blood for transfusion was often limited. When a patient needed blood, family members and friends had to donate, often in a short time. One of my physician friends trained at an indigent hospital in the South and said there was often very little blood available for transfusions. Often, no one wanted to donate blood, even to family members.

My doctor friend, while on the surgery service, cared for a patient who needed a transfusion. The family was approached, yet no one came forward. Then my friend "pulled the card" that always trumped everything. He told the family that if no one donated, Grandma would have to be transfused with dog's blood.

Six family members rose to their feet and walked to the blood bank donation area.

Practice, Practice, Practice

Infertility has plagued women since the book of Genesis. Mankind has struggled to find a way to have children and carry on the family name. Still, some women, even in the twenty-first century, remain childless. Modern technology has provided many the opportunity to conceive through sophisticated, albeit very costly, technology. My grandmother's approach was always to encourage those trying to conceive. Her motto was, "Practice, practice, practice!"

Bacterial Gorilla

A patient called me and said she had a discharge and could I call in some medication for her. I inquired about the discharge, and she said it was exactly like the last time when she had "bacterial gorilla."

I said, "What did you have?" and she repeated, "Bacterial gorilla." I told her she probably meant "bacterial vaginosis," and she said, "That's right—bacterial gorilla."

I suspected she meant bacterial gardnerella.

Sex Not Only Hurts but You Gain Weight

As a society, we struggle with encouraging our children to be abstinent and often fail. We talk to them about pregnancy and sexually transmitted diseases. I decided I needed to find something more compelling to steer my children away from premarital sex and convince them to wait. So I told my girls that sex hurts very badly and makes you gain weight (if you get pregnant).

I thought this had worked, at least with my younger daughter, until her first year of college. One Friday night at eleven p.m. I received a stat page to my daughter's cell phone. Thinking only the worst, I quickly dialed her number and she calmly answered.

She said, "First it was Santa Claus, then the Easter Bunny, and then the Tooth Fairy. You have lied to me again. Sex does not hurt!"

Just what I needed to hear on a Friday night.

Chief of Staff Called to Break Up Fight in Operating Room

The chief of staff is called on for many different situations. One particular morning, I was paged stat to the cesarean section room to break up a fight between the obstetrician and the pediatrician. The OB-GYN had cared for the baby until this point and had some idea of what should be done after delivery. The pediatrician thought to the contrary. So they decided to slug it out right there in the operating room in surgical gowns, masks, and gloves in front of the patient, family, and nurse anesthetist. I broke up the squabble and the surgery was done. Neither tolerated the other very well after that.

Watching the Sack Boys at Piggly Wiggly

During his first year of college, my son, Daniel, told me he wanted to be a doctor. We discussed the pros and cons. He had grown up the child of a physician, so practicing medicine was not a foreign idea. We discussed grades, MCAT (medical college admission test) scores, studying, etc. His grades were not good. He spent more time partying than studying.

Frustrated with him, I asked him to go for a ride with me to the local Piggly Wiggly, and we parked in front. We watched people coming and going and saw the sack boys carrying out their groceries. We just sat there for a while. Then my son asked me what we were doing, and I told him to watch the sack boys very carefully.

A short while later, Daniel asked, "Why are we doing this?"

I told him that if he did not study harder, not only was he not going to get into medical school, he was going to end up working as a sack boy.

His grades improved, and he got into medical school on his second attempt. He is now a third-year orthopedic surgery resident. Often, life has to be put into perspective.

Young Boy on Viagra

When Viagra came on the pharmaceutical market, it revolutionized the treatment of erectile dysfunction. Hugh Hefner at the Playboy Mansion announced that Viagra kept him going. There are a number of drugs in the class, all with similar action. Previous treatment of erectile dysfunction consisted of multiple injections around the base of the penis, vacuum devices, and herbal remedies.

I was completely unaware of other uses for this class of drugs, such as primary pulmonary hypertension. As a rural practitioner, I was always pleased to see patients I had cared for, along with their children.

One day, a mother brought in her young son, who looked great. She replied that he had been prescribed Viagra.

Without thinking, I replied, "Don't you think he's a little young for Viagra?"

She told me he was taking it for pulmonary hypertension.

I felt like an idiot!

Postpartum Patient Inquires about Eating the Placenta

As a country obstetrician, I have been asked many unusual questions over the years. I learned to be open-minded, as I never knew what to expect.

The first postpartum morning of a young girl I had delivered the night before asked if she really had to eat the placenta.

I said, "No—but who told you that?" I told her animals instinctively eat the placenta for the protein.

She said her grandmother told her she had to eat the placenta. I told her we threw the placentas away if they did not need to be sent to pathology. Her grandmother told her she had two choices: she could eat the placenta fried with hot mustard on it, or chopped up in spaghetti. She said her grandmother had told her if she did not eat it, the placenta would be disguised in her food.

I told her we did not do that.

Why Most Babies Seem to Be Born at Night

Among the great challenges of obstetrics and gynecology are the long hours and night work. A student on my service wanted to practice OB-GYN as a career but was dismayed because of the grueling hours. She became distressed after finding out the attending physician on call the night before did not get any sleep at all. Although the data is conflicted, it sure seems to me more babies are born at night.

A longtime patient of mine remarked recently that I looked tired and inquired about my sleep. She said she thought most babies were born at night, and I concurred. She asked me if I knew why that was, and I replied I didn't know.

She said, "Most babies are born at night because they are conceived at night."

I laughed and said, "That makes sense to me."

Strange Visitors at Church

All my life, I have been afraid of snakes. There are no nonpoisonous snakes. They all look alike and none of them are good. If I see one, I head in the other direction. When I moved to a rural area of Alabama, I had no idea that handling snakes was so popular in rural churches. I began to appreciate that such things happen, along with eating the placenta after a delivery. When invited to someone's church, I learned to ask if they handled snakes. If they did, I did not go anywhere near that church. They always said that if your faith in the Lord is good and you believe, the snakes will not bite you.

That seemed plausible until one of my friends, who was an emergency room physician, saw the pastor of one of these churches who had been bitten multiple times. Faith or no faith, snakes still bite. I understand that the snakes are passed down the pew at church much like the offering plate I was accustomed to. In the Baptist church, there is a Lord's Supper table sitting in front of the pulpit, which has the offering plate and flowers sitting on it if no communion is planned for that day. However, if something resembling your mother's cedar chest is in front of the pulpit, don't go near it. It is the snake box!

Called to Deliver Octuplets—Next Door

I was working in my front yard one day when I heard the children next door running across the yard to me. They were holding their cat above their heads. They asked me if their cat was going to have kittens. She was very pregnant and I could feel several kittens inside her abdomen. Part of rural OB-GYN training includes prenatal care of pets.

Several days later, the phone rang and it was the children next door. They said, "Come quick! Our cat is delivering!"

Sure enough, the tired mother cat was delivering the last of her eight kittens when I arrived. Sorry, no delivery charges because I missed the delivery! She licked the kittens clean and ate the placenta, which most of my patients generally don't do!

Patient Asks for a Prescription for Ecstasy

Obstetrician and gynecologists serve as the primary-care providers for 65 percent of the women in the United States. They often write prescriptions for more than just OB-GYN medications but usually stay away from prescribing addictive drugs such as narcotics and benzodiazepines for non-OB-GYN uses. Patients occasionally ask for prescriptions for new drugs they see on television, hear about, or read about in magazines.

One morning in an outlying clinic, I saw a longtime patient who was suffering with postmenopausal symptoms we were trying to treat. The worst symptom was a decreased interest in sex. We had tried everything I knew or could find out about. On this morning, she asked me to write her a prescription for ecstasy. I was speechless. I told her that was an illegal drug. She told me she thought it was okay with a prescription.

I said, "Of all people, you should know better, since you work for the sheriff's office in the drug task force division."

Winfield Cafeteria: "That Is All You Need to Eat"

Most hospitals today, large and small, have cafeterias. That was certainly the case in the rural hospital where I practiced at the time. I ate every lunch there, many breakfasts, and occasionally at night when I was on call. I got to know the staff, and they got to knew me. They would call me when they were serving food I liked. Over time, I noticed one of the women on the serving line always gave me less food than everyone else.

One day, they were serving food I really liked and my portions were tiny. That did it. I asked her why I got such small portions, expecting the problem to be corrected with an apology.

To my amazement, she replied," That is all you need to eat!"

Mother Delivers Ten-Pound Baby at Home and Needs Suturing

Pam had delivered her first baby in the hospital, but the rest were delivered at home. She and her family did not have health insurance. After much prayer, they decided on a home delivery but wanted prenatal care until about thirty-two weeks. She saw one of my partners and received regular care until thirty-two weeks but then disappeared from the face of the earth. Her OB-GYN could not find her or anything about her. Her husband was an ultrasonographer, and he did check the baby periodically by ultrasound. At forty weeks she went into labor, which was long because the baby was large. She delivered a healthy ten-pound baby without anesthesia.

The delivery was complicated by massive bleeding and a fourth-degree perineal tear into the rectum. The bleeding finally slowed, but the tears needed repairing, so her husband called the obstetrician they had not seen in eight weeks. The husband explained she needed sewing up. The OB-GYN said for them to get the doctor who'd delivered her baby to sew her up. The husband told the doctor he had delivered the baby. Again, the OB-GYN said for them to let the doctor who'd delivered sew her up.

So she didn't get sewn up, and she healed with gaping tears. She came to see me six weeks later, but it was too late to repair.

Testicles in Mammogram Machine

I saw one of my dear patients for a yearly checkup. I recommended she have a mammogram. She complained that the machine squeezed on her breasts so bad they hurt. She said, "I'll tell you what. You put your testicles in the mammogram machine, and if they don't hurt, I'll put my breasts in and have a mammogram!"

"The Two Best Things Are Great Sex and a Stat Section"

The middle of my career was spent in a small rural town in Alabama. It was a new hospital that offered good pay, state-of-the-art equipment, and three partners. The hospital served a draw area of one hundred fifty thousand people in West Alabama. During the course of working there, I gradually met all those I worked with. Everyone was pleasant and worked well together. One particular nurse said she liked stat sections because of the excitement, and I concurred. She said, "In fact, the two best things in life are great sex and a stat section for distress." I really did not know what to say.

Dirty Gloves Thrown into Patient's Purse

Gloves are worn for every procedure in our office. After one use they are thrown into the garbage container lined with a red hazardous-material liner. One day, a patient laid her open purse by the garbage container. As I took off my gloves, I accidentally threw the gloves into her purse. Fortunately, they were not soiled, and I took them out and apologized.

"Cocktail Style or Sunday School Style?"

I have taken care of patients for thirty-four years, and after visiting and interviewing patients, I have always given them a gown and sheet to put on for the examination. I explain which is which, and how to put them on.

On one occasional, before I could explain how to put on the gown and sheet, the patient said as I handed her the items, "Cocktail style or Sunday school style?"

I asked, "What?"

She repeated her question. I asked her to explain.

She said, "If it opens in the front, it has a plunging neckline like a cocktail dress—or cocktail style. If it opens in the back so the neckline is high in the front and the plunge is in the back, it would be like you were going to Sunday school—or Sunday school style. You would never wear a plunging neckline to Sunday school."

Check Warts on Penis at Family Reunion

The family reunion is a great medical experience. It is an opportunity to hear about everyone's illnesses, their interpretation of their illnesses, and everyone's response. It is, however, rare for a male relative to pull out his penis to show you his warts. But it happened. We at least went indoors, and he showed me in private a penis covered with warts. I was dumbfounded! As a physician, I have come to appreciate that it is unusual for men to have warts that are visible. But he did.

I convinced him to come to my office, and we spent the afternoon cutting off the warts. There was one large pedunculated (elongated and stalk-like) wart about mid-shaft on the top. He told me not to cut it off because all his girlfriends like that one very much. I left it alone. We went back to the family reunion—but I was no longer hungry. He called me the next day and said he was so sore he could not go to work.

Is ED at Your House?

Retired men often get together in the mornings at local fast food restaurants, eat breakfast, drink coffee, and talk about the old times. The talks could be on any topic. A common statement was, "Is ED at your house?" In fact, the statement was mentioned most days.

I thought maybe one of their friends was named "Ed." Finally, I asked, "Who is Ed?"

Laughing, they replied, "Erectile dysfunction. ED comes to most of our houses. He has visited most of us. He will eventually come to your house."

"Do I Look Better with My Clothes On or Off?"

I had taken care of this certain patient for years and knew her well. She was a good friend of my wife. She was well-off and well-to-do. She was sixty-five years old and very pleasant. She always came to the office well-dressed.

Her well-woman visit was no different from any other. We talked, I examined her with a nurse, and I left for her to get dressed.

As she left, she said, "Do I look better with my clothes on or off?"

I was stunned. I finally said, "You always look very nice."

She said thanks and left.

Woman Delivers Baby in Emergency Department Restroom

Half the counties in Alabama have no obstetric provider. It is not unusual for a pregnant woman to present to an emergency department whose hospital does not have obstetric services. Sometimes patients know they are pregnant, and others claim they did not notice they were term pregnant. Some of these women have such advanced dilatation they cannot be transferred, according to the EMTALA (Emergency Medical Treatment and Active Labor Act) rules.

One such patient presented to the ER. Before she could be checked, she felt pelvic pressure and went to the restroom thinking she needed to have a bowel movement. She delivered a healthy, seven-pound male infant into the commode. She rang the emergency button and the nurse pulled the infant out of the toilet.

The patient named the new baby John.

Woman Has Terrible Vulvar Itching

Gynecologists take vulvar itching seriously because it can be one of the earliest signs of vulvar cancer.

One patient presented with vulvar itching. I questioned her about it at length and asked the usual detailed questions.

Finally, she said, "It itched so bad I thought I was going to have to call in the neighbors to help me scratch."

That sounded pretty serious!

Woman Has Open Laparotomy and Drives Home

A woman I had cared for for many years needed surgery to remove her ovaries. We went through the whole informed-consent process in which I explained how long the surgery would last and how long she would need to be in the hospital.

The case went well. During surgery, a full-length, midline incision for exploratory was utilized, extending from the umbilicus to the pubic hairline.

After I dictated the surgical note, I went to the recovery room to check on her, but she was not there. I asked the nurse about her whereabouts, and she said the patient had been in her bed in the recovery room just a few minutes ago and was doing fine. She did not smoke, so there was no need for her to go outside.

We couldn't find her. I called her on her cell phone, and she answered. I said, "Where are you? I've looked all over for you. I was worried."

She said she was doing fine and decided to just go home rather than stay in the hospital. So she pulled out her IV line, got dressed, and drove home.

I asked her to come back to the hospital, and she said she didn't need to. She said she would call me if she needed anything.

I did get her to let me call in some oral Lortab in case she was in any pain. I saw her a week later and she was fine.

My Son Asked What Breast Implants Feel Like

The world of plastic surgery has invaded high schools. Many high school girls have had breast reductions and augmentation mammoplasty. If they feel their breasts are too large, they want them smaller. If they believe their breasts are too small, they want them enlarged.

My children know if they need me urgently, such as in an emergency, they page me and put in a special code so that I recognize it and call back as soon as possible.

Late one Friday night, I received a stat page identified by a code from my son. I called him immediately. He greeted me and asked me what breast implants feel like. Realizing this to be unusual, and not seeming to be an emergency, I asked him why he wanted to know. He said one of the girls in his class had recently had breast implants. She was telling my son about them, knowing he was interested in going to medical school.

Believe me, nothing like this ever happened to me in high school.

He told me she was going to take him upstairs and let him see and feel her implants. So why did he call me? He wanted some idea of what they actually felt like. He was anxious to have this data, especially since he wanted to go to medical school.

I asked him if he had a condom with him, but he said he didn't. I said in that case, he'd better not go upstairs to see her breasts and should take her word for it.

He said he didn't understand. I told him that one day he would.

Office under a Swimming Pool

Rural OB-GYN was great, and my practice grew quickly. In a short time, I needed a larger space, but space was hard to obtain, especially right at the hospital where I needed to be to labor patients and be able to be in the office at the same time.

The administrator notified me he had found me some good office space. In fact, it was on the ground floor of the new fitness center, which was on campus. There were plenty of exam rooms, plenty of parking, storage, a large front office, and an expanded waiting room.

I asked, "What's the catch?"

He said, "It's underneath the Olympic-size swimming pool."

I asked about leaking, and he said there had not been any. Still, it was an uncomfortable thought being under the swimming pool.

Space was short, so I moved in. It was quite nice and spacious. The rent was reasonable. Everything went well for a while.

One Sunday, I needed a patient's chart. As I opened the front door, the water was six inches deep. I am uncertain why there wasn't more water. It was an awful feeling.

IX

Practicing at the School of Medicine in Tuscaloosa

The final chapter in my life appears to be about practicing medicine at the University of Alabama School of Medicine in Tuscaloosa, Alabama. What an honor! I applied to be a faculty member four times over my career before being accepted. The first time was just out of residency, and the chair told me he had filled all vacant position the day before.

The second time I applied, the faculty had dwindled down to one physician. My private practice partner and I, both graduates of the program, were concerned about the department surviving. We both applied and guaranteed that one of us would always be there during a twenty-four-hour shift. We proposed providing the service free for six months. After that period of time, we could negotiate faculty membership. The dean never responded to us.

The third application went well, but the credentialing secretary at the hospital would not give me the staff application because I did not live there. I told her that if granted staff privileges, I would move there. She still refused because I had to live there first.

The fourth application was a charm, and I became a faculty member and have been there ever since.

Nurse Practitioner Rotation and the Chancellor's Secretary

One afternoon, a nurse practitioner student who had made an appointment with me came for an interview. She was doing her last rotation before graduation and needed a clinical experience in

OB-GYN. She asked for a specific date, but we unfortunately were full and at our maximum for nurse practitioner students, with more than the usual number of medical students, residents, and fellows. She started crying, and I felt bad.

Then came the kicker. She said, "My mother is the executive secretary for the chancellor of the University of Alabama Education System. I went to see her yesterday, and while talking about the situation, the chancellor walked in. He heard the conversation and told me to come to the medical school and ask for Dr. Dan Avery, who he was sure could help me."

I said, "He is correct. Do you want to start this afternoon or wait until tomorrow morning?" My mother did not raise a fool!

Patient Talks on Cell Phone during Pelvic Examination

Despite all the signs in our clinic to turn off cell phones, many patients still use them while we're trying to talk to them. Some even talk simultaneously. I had a patient who talked continuously while I was trying to interview and examine her—including during the pelvic exam. It was aggravating. While I was doing the speculum exam, she said her husband wanted to know how everything looked. I replied that everything was normal. Then she said her husband wanted me to take a picture of the inside of her vagina with her cell phone camera. I refused.

Patient Dehisces and Fills Abdomen with Toilet Paper

An eighty-five-year-old woman showed up at our regional campus office with vaginal bleeding. She had never had a pap smear. I found a large lesion on her cervix. Biopsy revealed an invasive squamous cell carcinoma. She was referred to a GYN oncologist at our main campus. She was a candidate for a radical hysterectomy with pelvic and periaortic lymph node dissections. She actually did well and went home in five days.

Ten days later she called and said her incision had "come undone." She was informed to immediately come to the emergency department. Four or five hours passed before she arrived.

Our service was consulted to see her. She had completely dehisced (ruptured) and had spent hours filling her abdominal cavity with several rolls of toilet paper to absorb the fluid. Upon examination, she was literally full of toilet paper. She was transferred to the GYN oncology service forty-five miles away at the main campus. It took the oncology service twenty minutes to close the incision but five hours to pick out all the toilet paper.

Sunday School Teacher Brings Lesson on Ethics

One Sunday morning before announcements, a member of my Sunday school class, whom I knew well, told me about his bicycle accident the day before. He was riding with his sons and trying to "outdo" them. During the course of a race, he went off the road and injured multiple areas of his body, including his right flank. He did not go to the doctor.

From years of experience, I knew where this was heading. He then asked me to write him a prescription for twenty Lortab 10s.

Surprised, I said, "You're not my patient, and I cannot write controlled-substance prescriptions for you."

He responded that he had been to my practice and saw someone who sees men. He said he would ask another physician he knew.

Ironically, the regular Sunday school teacher was out, and this person had agreed to teach the class that day.

Guess what the lesson was on?

"Ethics and ethical behavior."

"A Neighbor Checked Me, and I Am Six Centimeters Dilated"

Obstetric patients regularly call to report contractions and ask if they need to come to the hospital. One night, a patient called and said she was six centimeters dilated and hurting with contractions.

I said, "Of course you need to come to the hospital if you are six centimeters dilated. How do you know how much you are dilated?"

She said, "A neighbor checked me, and he said I was six centimeters." She said he knew what he was doing. When she got to the labor room, she was indeed six centimeters dilated.

New Treatment for Postmenopausal Symptoms

Patients are always looking for new treatments for common maladies. For many, life begins at forty but hot flashes start at fifty. One of my postmenopausal patients related to me that she had developed a new treatment for hot flashes. She said that while driving her car, she pulls her skirt or dress up over the steering wheel. She holds the steering wheel covered by clothing, which allows her to cool down her body with the cool air from the air conditioner. I told her I hope she drives alone.

"Do You Have an Anatomy Picture of the Vagina?"

During the course of practicing medicine, you see and hear everything. I saw a patient with dyspareunia (painful intercourse). She brought her unwilling husband to the office. He remained very quiet during the entire visit. He had a vested interest in her visit because it involved his ability to get sex. His wife went through a long explanation of why she did not want sex.

At the end of the visit, the husband finally spoke and asked me if I had an anatomy book. I said I did. He asked if the book had an anatomical picture of the vagina. I again said yes. He asked me if I would make him a copy of the picture of the vagina. I said I would and asked him why. He said he did not want to forget what a vagina looked like!

Dean Suggests I Run Obstetric Clinic at Mental Institution

From time to time, most mental institutions admit women who are pregnant. The number is so few, however, that even large institutions do not routinely have obstetricians on staff but contract out the service. Most of the obstetricians in Tuscaloosa have at one time or another provided care to mental institutions, all with regret of the terrible mess they often found themselves in. The patients are disruptive in the office and the waiting room and often drive other patients away. Some patients, staff, and even physicians are afraid of the pregnant mental patients. One of the largest mental hospitals in Tuscaloosa needed a consulting obstetrician, but no one wanted the job.

The attorney from the mental hospital was a member of the medical school board of directors. She asked the dean of the medical school to help her secure an obstetrician. The dean asked me to ask the physicians in our department if they would provide the service. Of course they balked.

But sometimes authority figures can explain things in a more meaningful way when they have not heard the answer they want. The dean explained to me that the university was trying to buy the mental hospital, and it would help if the medical school provided this much-needed service. Still I declined.

Then the dean made it very clear. He said, "Dan, you're up for both promotion and tenure. Your promotion materials are on my desk. I am the person who makes the final decision."

I asked him when he wanted me to start the clinic at the mental hospital.

He said, "Wednesday."

Caught Speeding by the Mental Health Hospital Police

All doctors and nurses have stories about getting stopped by law enforcement for speeding. Most of the time, unless the speed limit exceeded is egregious, we are given a warning and no ticket. We are usually given the standard warning not to speed, and we ease by until the next time we break the law.

There is some personal reward in whom you are chased and caught by for speeding. Our highest respect goes to the Alabama State Troopers, etc., but being stopped by the hospital security guards seems way down on the list.

One afternoon I was driving on the mental hospital campus to the medical building when I noticed a police car behind me, its red and blue lights flashing. Since I was just easing along, I pulled over to let him pass. I stopped right in front of the medical building where I saw patients. To my surprise, he pulled right behind me. Knowing I was not speeding, I wondered what he wanted with me.

As he approached, I rolled down my window. I said, "Can I help you?"

He said, "You were speeding."

"How fast was I going?"

"I clocked you at fifteen miles per hour."

I asked, "Fifty or fifteen?"

"Fifteen."

I asked, "What's the speed limit?"

He said, "Five miles per hour," and pointed to an old rusty sign.

I said, "I'm unsure if my car will go that slow."

"What are you doing here?" he asked.

"I'm a doctor and take care of the pregnant patients here."

He said, "I'm not going to give you a ticket this time, but don't speed anymore. You might run over a patient. Go on to the clinic."

The next time I went to the Bryce Clinic, the nurses greeted me, saying, "Today is your lucky day. The police car is broken down!"

Placenta Has Hair on It

The number of patients in labor at any one time is unpredictable. On this particular day, the medical school teaching service had four women in labor. As luck would have it, three were ready to deliver at the same time. The first patient was a "walk-in" with no prenatal care who weighed more than five hundred pounds. I checked her cervix on admission and she was ready to deliver. I helped two medical students do the delivery, and the baby did well. I left them to deliver the placenta.

Next I went to the second room, where the patient was crowning and the baby was quickly out. I left the resident to finish up. Then I went to the third room for the delivery, and in no more than a few minutes the head was out.

I was paged back to the first room, where the students said the placenta had hair on it. Sure enough, the patient had twins, and the students eased out the second baby with no problem. I put on long gloves and checked for a third baby, but there were only two.

The two students never appreciated that they had delivered vaginal twins, which few residents get to do.

Summoning the University Police to Tow Away the Dean's RV

College football is a major interest in the South and especially at the University of Alabama, where it almost approaches a religious experience. The University of Alabama is located in Tuscaloosa, Alabama, a town of about one hundred thousand people. On football game weekends, an extra hundred thousand people crowd into Tuscaloosa. The traffic is bumper to bumper, and parking can be scarce. To help the parking situation, the university allows all their parking lots to be utilized for game weekend parking. The restriction is that outside parking in those lots cannot begin until six on Friday night and must end by noon on Sunday. There are always a few offenders.

One Friday morning I came to work early, probably around six. I'm usually the first to arrive at the school of medicine, and sometimes I drive around the building to see what's going on and who's there.

Lo and behold, there was a relatively new, burgundy-colored RV parked in the front of the medical school, taking up half a dozen parking spaces. I was stunned and immediately called the university police to report the infraction and ask them to have the RV towed away. During the call, I was paged stat to labor and delivery to attend to an emergency cesarean section. I was in the process of giving the dispatcher the location of the RV but told her I had to go to a delivery and would call her back afterward.

The C-section went well, with a healthy mother and baby. But the labor rooms were full and the service busy. I forgot about the RV. Later that morning I made it back to the medical school. I went in and spoke to the departmental secretary.

She casually said, "Did you see the dean's new RV in front of the building?"

I felt faint and dizzy. I had chest pain and had to sit down.

She asked, "What in the world is wrong?"

I told her, and she thought it was hilarious. I told her not to say anything to anybody. Everyone I passed started laughing when they saw me. I had a pretty good idea she had not kept the information to herself.

I was uncertain whether I should starting packing my office or go to the dean and apologize. I saw my academic career pass in front of my eyes. I saw myself cutting grass on a riding lawnmower or being the greeter at Walmart. Eventually, those feelings thankfully went away.

I no longer summon the police for any parking violations. I look the other way when I see an RV.

The following spring the graduating class of medical students asked me to be the commencement speaker at the honors convocation. Of course I was honored and accepted. My speech focused on enjoying the practice of medicine, being honest with patients, and giving good care—and I mentioned the incident with the dean's RV. Everyone laughed like they had never heard this story, but I knew they probably had.

Everything went okay until the time came for the dean to give out awards. He began by asking his wife to go outside and make sure I had not called the police to tow away their car. The responding laughter raised the roof. I would have crawled under the table if I was not so large. Unfortunately, I was sitting at the front table *by the dean's wife.* She'd thought the whole RV ordeal was funny; the dean did not.

How to Get a Physician to the Telephone Immediately

Often, one of the most challenging problems for a physician is getting a colleague on the phone. You have to go through practically everyone who works there just to reach a fellow physician.

So I came up with an idea, and it has always been foolproof. When I call a fellow physician's office, I say, "This is so and so with the IRS.

I'm calling about a delinquent tax payment. I need to come by and pick up a check from Dr. so and so."

It always works! The first time, physicians are mad at me but are relieved it's really not the IRS! Over the years, most of those close to me know it's me. But it still works!

"Doctor, Our Baby Looks Exactly Like You"

I called a longtime friend and colleague and told his receptionist the following. I made up a fake name and said, "Dr. Denson delivered our baby." I told her mother and baby were doing fine. But, I said, the older the baby got, the more it looked like Dr. Denson. I asked, "Could Dr. Denson possibly the father of the baby?"

There was a long pause. The receptionist said I would need to talk to the nurse. I relayed the same story, and she too was speechless. She said I would need to talk to Dr. Denson.

Before I could finish the first sentence, Dr. Denson recognized my voice and said he would get me back very soon—when I least expected it.

"From the Womb to the Tomb"

I am often teased about the many jobs I've had since I was fifteen and on my own. I've gotten to do a lot of things and have had many great life experiences. My dad died after a lengthy illness when I was a teenager, and my mother was very sick and went to live with our grandmother. My younger brother and I lived in our house in West End in Tuscaloosa. I worked in a funeral home. After going to medical school and completing residency training in pathology, I switched to the other end of life and did an OB-GYN residency. My colleagues thought I'd covered the spectrum of life and my motto should be "From the womb to the tomb—I will care for all your needs!"

Special Treatment for Kidney Stones

I've had a number of kidney stones over my adult years; so had my dad. My wife never had any.

One Sunday while driving home after church, my wife started taking off her clothes. This was an unusual occurrence, but I didn't say anything.

When she got down to her bra and panties, I said, "You know it's daylight and someone is going to see you, right? By the way—what in the world are you doing?"

These are the things that husbands dream about. However, it does not usually occur in the daytime, especially after church.

She said she was hurting very badly.

I said where and she said the left lower quadrant. I asked, "Have you ever had stones?"

She said no, and I asked what it felt like. She said, "I don't know."

When we got home, she got out of my SUV in our driveway in her bra and panties. She went into the house and urinated blood, so we thought she had a kidney stone. She took some pain medication and finally passed a sizable renal stone. She quickly felt better.

However, I am unclear how taking all of her clothes off helped.

Very Large Scrubs Are in the Back

There are several uniform stores in Tuscaloosa, Alabama, that sell medical scrubs. Since there are several hospitals and many doctor's offices, scrubs are a big business. I went in and asked for scrubs in size 3X.

In a loud voice, the clerk replied that very large-sized scrubs are in the back of the store. I was embarrassed and sheepishly looked around to see if I knew anyone there; fortunately, I did not.

I went to the back and saw the few scrubs the store had. I started to just look around the store, and the clerk at the front hollered at me and said, "I said the very large sizes were in the back."

I looked through the clothes, and she appeared behind me. I said, "Are there any red scrubs in 3X?"

She said, "There are only a few colors in very large sizes."

I left. About a month later, I returned to the store. It was full of people I worked with at the hospital.

Right off, this same clerk yelled, "Very large sizes are in the back!"

Someone Else Is in My Call Bed

Obstetric call can be brutal. Sometimes you get very little sleep and occasionally no sleep at all. Sleep is at a premium.

One night I got everyone delivered and the labor board was clean. It was time to get some sleep. I was exhausted. I went to the call room but did not turn the light on because I knew the room like the back of my hand. I slipped my scrub shirt off and left on my scrub pants.

I slid right into the call bed to find someone else already there. I thought, *This is just great. Someone has stolen where I was going to sleep.*

I slid out of bed and cracked the door open. I could see our obstetric fellow in my bed. I put my shirt back on and eased out the door. The fellow never woke up, and I hope he never knew I had gotten into bed with him.

History and Physical before Knee Replacement

My orthopedic surgeon told me I needed a total knee replacement. I went to the scheduling office to make the final arrangements.

While we were there, a physician assistant arrived and said she was supposed to perform my history and physical. I asked when and she said she could do it while the secretary was doing the scheduling arrangements. I thought this was a little odd. At my clinic, we put patients in an exam room, ask them to undress, and ask a lot of questions before doing an exam. She did none of this.

She asked if my medications had changed and I said no.

She said, "Okay—that's your history and physical."

I asked if she needed to listen to my heart and lungs, and she said no. I asked if she could tell whether I had situs inversus (a congenital condition in which the organs of the chest and abdomen are arranged in a perfect mirror image reversal of the normal positioning), and she said no.

She asked if I had situs inversus, and I said no.

So how good do you think that history and physical was for someone who actually has a number of health problems?

Medical Student Rides Bicycle to Delivery across Town

Robert was a great medical student. He was always well-prepared, courteous, and gracious. He was well-liked by his peers and certainly by the clinic staff.

Our faculty covered the labor rooms at two separate hospitals. Robert was assigned to Dr. Reed, and most of his deliveries were at Northport Medical Center, about five miles away.

Robert lived in Alberta City, two miles from the medical school and main teaching hospital. But Robert was not making it to deliveries on time. I asked him about missing the deliveries, and he told me he was riding his bicycle to the hospitals when it was not raining. That worked out when the delivery was at the main hospital because it was two blocks from the medical school and one mile from his house.

The deliveries in Northport were the problem because the hospital there was five miles away. He was riding his bicycle in rush-hour traffic or he had to ride his bicycle to Alberta City, get his car, and then drive to Northport.

I suggested he drive his car when he was on call.

Resident Lacerates Attending's Hand during Cesarean Section

Steve wanted to become an obstetrics fellow. During his senior year as a resident, he assisted at cesarean sections to gain as much experience as possible before his fellowship year. He and Dr. Hooper had a repeat cesarean section scheduled. I was in the process of completing an outpatient surgical procedure when I was paged stat to labor and delivery. I immediately called the labor room and was told Dr. Hooper needed me stat in the cesarean section room! On opening the door to the section room, blood was everywhere, but the patient had not yet been incised. The blood was coming from Dr. Hooper, who was holding his hand wrapped in a surgical towel, blood dripping from it.

He told me Steve had accidentally cut his hand as they were starting the cesarean section. I told Dr. Hooper to go to the emergency department for stitches. I did the cesarean section with the residents.

As I went back to outpatient surgery to do my next case, the charge nurse said they were holding room 2 for the plastic surgeon to explore Dr. Hooper's hand because they thought ligaments had been lacerated. Dr. Hooper was sewn up and in a month was doing fine. Nobody wanted to operate with Steve.

A few days later, Steve asked me if cutting Dr. Hooper would affect his chances of becoming a fellow, and I said, "Probably."

Sitting in Spilled Betadine in the Operating Room

Until recently, Betadine was the preparation of choice for gynecologic and most other surgical cases. If left on for a prolonged period of time, Betadine is toxic to the skin. It also stains everything. I had a dilatation and curettage/hysteroscopy case in the outpatient operating room. As requested, Betadine was used to prep the vagina. Unfortunately, some of the Betadine spilled on the stool I sit on to do vaginal surgery. Not noticing it, I sat in it. It was not enough to feel anything, but it left a two-inch diameter brown spot in the center of my buttocks. Not knowing it was there, I wore those scrubs all day. Guess what everyone thought.

Medical Student Goes Home On Call

Labor and delivery was busy, as we had four deliveries before midnight. Everyone was tired after a long day at the clinic and the regular call responsibilities with four vaginal deliveries. As we were writing delivery notes and signing orders, the medical student announced that since we were all there and work was caught up, he would cut the call night short and go home.

He said, "Just call me if you need me and I'll come back."
One can imagine how this went over with the residents.

Dr. Jones Is the Father of the Baby

My longtime partner, Dr. Jones, and I were seeing patients during clinic one afternoon. Emily, his nurse, pulled me aside and asked if I would see one of Dr. Jones's patients. I said I would. She said it was an infertility patient who was now pregnant. She had been seeing Dr. Jones since he was in Atlanta years ago and had followed him to Tuscaloosa. I said that was okay.

Emily then told me Dr. Jones was the father of the baby.

I said, "Wait a minute. What do you mean?"

Emily said the patient had never been able to get pregnant, so Dr. Jones just fathered the baby.

I thought, *I can do this.* So I went into the room and introduced myself.

The couple was cordial. We listened to heart tones and measured the fundus. Everything checked out okay.

Then I said, "I understand y'all are from Atlanta."

They replied they were from Mexico.

I said, "How long have you known Dr. Jones?"

They replied they'd met him about two months ago.

I'd been had.

As I walked out of the room, Emily and Dr. Jones were rolling on the floor, hysterically laughing.

I told them they were up and their time was coming very soon.

"Come On Home, I'm in the Bed"

During the course of the work day, Dr. Hooper and I changed offices. Changing offices also meant a change of telephones and voice mail. We didn't think much about it, and the day went on as usual.

Toward the end of the day, he was going through his voice mail. He immediately became quiet and said, "Dan, I think this call is for you."

I said, "Why do you think that?"

He told me to listen to the message. My wife had called me, which is not uncommon, and she'd left me a message.

Unfortunately, it was on Dr. Hooper's voice mail.

The message said, "Come on home. I've had a shower and am in bed waiting for you."

My wife would not show her face at our office for six months after that.

Giant Funny Spells (GFS)

Having spent almost half my career practicing full-time or part-time in rural Alabama I came across a term in a medical record called a "giant funny spell," or GFS. It was described as "a fit-like activity, followed by passing out." These fits usually occurred at church in the afternoon after a prolonged worship service with dinner to follow at the church. After the patient passed out, he or she would be rushed to the hospital emergency department poised as either syncope (fainted) or a seizure. Seizure was easy to exclude because the patient would open his or her eyes and talk to you rationally and was not postictal (that "fuzzy period" after a patient has had a seizure). The patient certainly did not urinate or defecate in his or her undergarments. Workup, labs, and imaging were always normal. After some rest, the patient was ready to leave. The diagnosis would be "giant funny spell." There is no CPT or ICD-9 (codes used for billing and charting) for "GFS," so medical records will no longer allow that diagnosis on the chart.

Medical Student Cosigns Resident's Note

Medical students appear first on the wards very early in the morning and start seeing patients and writing notes. Next, interns show up and do pretty much the same. This is followed by residents, and finally the fellows, who supervise the service. Attendings may or may not write a note but always cosign all notes for everyone.

One student just could not get up in the mornings, and he even slept through rounds one weekday morning. This particular morning he was very late—in fact, it was almost time for morning report where the patients on our service would be discussed. He did not have time to write any notes, so he just wrote below the resident notes: "Agree with above."

I have never seen that done in thirty years.

Aunt Wants Vagina Checked at Family Reunion

After residency training, family reunions were an opportunity for my family to get free medical advice. Aunt Ruth told me something was hanging out of her vagina. She asked me to look at whatever it was. I suggested we look at her in my office rather than at the family reunion.

Potato Pessaries

I learned from my grandmother that "necessity is the mother of invention." This was a saying I'd always heard, but she explained it in a way I could understand. She was a bit more open after I graduated from medical school. I had learned about pessaries (a removable device inserted in the vagina to support a prolapsed organ) in medical school, but my knowledge was limited. Before commercial pessaries, women used potatoes to support the bladder. They could be trimmed to fit and even sized again later. The only problem was that with the moisture in the vagina, the potato sprouted, and green sprouts would grow out of the vagina. The green sprouts would periodically have to be trimmed.

Department Chair Has Dermatology Appointment with Student

In our town, there is a group of eight dermatologists and a single other practitioner, all of whom are very busy. It is difficult to get an appointment with the group, and emergency visits are unheard of. My wife runs the university's student health service. On October 12 she called for an urgent appointment for a terrible rash. She was told the next appointment was in mid-January 2011.

I recently called my regular dermatologist for an appointment. I have been a patient of the group for thirty-five years. I was told there were no available appointments, but I could see a medical student in the student teaching clinic. As a department chair at the medical school in town, I was not thrilled but was willing to do so. My concern was that a medical student may not know any more than I would. I had practiced medicine for nearly thirty years and had completed residency training in both pathology and OB-GYN.

When I got to their office, I was quickly seen by a staff dermatologist.

Falling Down Steps after Knee Replacement

Nearing sixty years old, my knee cartilage was completely destroyed. I could hardly walk and often fell. My orthopedic surgeon had told me I would know when it was time to replace it. It was time. I hated being a patient; it is always more fun to be a caregiver than the care receiver. The knee was replaced and surgery went well. But then it was time to go home, and I could hardly walk. We got tucked into my truck and headed home.

Everything was okay until the garage door went up. There stood my biggest nightmare for the next two months—the steps. How would I get into the house? I crawled up the steps into the house and pulled up onto a chair and then a wheelchair.

As I learned to use crutches, I decided to walk up a ramp a friend loaned us. I got halfway up the steps, lost my balance, and rolled down the lower steps. I hit the garage floor and rolled up under my truck.

All my wife could do was laugh. She said, "You weigh 260 pounds, and I couldn't catch you anyway!"

She did help snake me out from under the truck when she quit laughing.

Ceiling Falls in Call Room

Labor and delivery was in the old part of the hospital. In fact, it was so old that it was much like it was when I was born. The call rooms were small and hot, but they were situated close to labor and delivery. The ceiling in the call room leaked right over the bed. The usual scenario was that a physician would be woken by water dripping on him or her during the night. Finally, the physician would wake up and move somewhere else. This went on for about six months.

One night I woke to more dripping than there had ever been. I turned the light on. The ceiling was pouring water and just about to fall on me. Finally it collapsed, and water went everywhere.

The next morning the hospital engineer told me it was the commode leaking on me from the cardiovascular surgery waiting room above me. I thought, *What great news . . . a commode has been dripping on me at night for six months.*

Sitting on the Toilet Doing Medical Records

From April to July each year we have an extra group of medical students. There are fourth years, old third years, and new third years. There are people everywhere. There are not enough seats, computers, and even work areas. I needed to complete and sign charts, but there was nowhere to sit. I noticed an empty restroom and sat on the commode to use my tablet PC. There was no reason to shut the door because I was dressed. It caused a lot of attention and pictures. I suspect those pictures will show up at a later time, when I least expect it. But I got my charts done.

My Wife's White Cotton Suit and Syncope at the First Baptist Church

I joined the medical school faculty in Tuscaloosa, Alabama, in 2003. My wife, who is a nurse of many years, and I started attending the First Baptist Church. We usually went to the early morning Sunday service because it was traditional—that is, women wore dresses, men wore suits, old hymns were sung, etc. There was no rock-type music or smoke in the air, and the invocation was not played with drums and electric guitars but on a pipe organ. Most older people were like us; they went to the early service.

We sat in the back row since I was usually on call. The first Sunday an elderly lady collapsed near the front of the sanctuary, and several men carried her out. Shortly after that, I felt someone tapping my shoulder, and a deacon said they needed me in the area outside the sanctuary. As I got up to leave, my wife just sat there. I told her to come with me. Now who do you think is more comfortable managing a resuscitation, an OB-GYN or a forty-year veteran ICU nurse? Please!

The next Sunday was right before Christmas. During the special choral music, the choir director collapsed and started seizing. To be honest, I was not paying attention and was looking around. It caught my attention when everyone stood up because it was not a usual time to stand. The same deacon again tapped me on my shoulder and said I had better just go on down to the front of the church where the choir director was seizing. I walked up on the platform, and about twenty people were staring at him—along with an ophthalmologist, a CRNA (a certified registered nurse anesthetist), and me.

He quit seizing and was transported to the hospital via ambulance. One of the church members was an attorney who ran down the hall with an automatic defibrillator and wanted to use it on the choir director. I stopped him since I did not think it would help.

We discovered a pattern. When my wife wore a white cotton suit, someone collapsed at church. When she wore something else, no one collapsed.

The next Sunday she wore her white cotton suit, and an older gentleman collapsed near the back of the church. I was more attentive this time and got up so I would not have to be summoned. Three men and I carried this man to the foyer where my wife and I could attend him. A retired internist showed up to help this time. When the unconscious gentleman came around, he said he received his care at the medical school by one of the internists down the hall from me. He was transported to the hospital.

We decided that for everyone's health she would quit wearing the white cotton suit. We ended up going to another Baptist church across town, but she did not wear the white suit.

One Sunday they asked us if we wanted to be on the code team for certain services. They had nice equipment to use. I suppose there was a member in that church who also wore white cotton suits.

Are You Sexually Active?

The sexual history is an important part of an OB-GYN history and physical. Medical students and residents are trained in tactfully asking questions about sexual interest, sexual partners, sexually transmitted diseases, penile discharge, contraception, and dyspareunia (painful intercourse).

This history usually begins with, "Are you sexually active?"

Patients usually reply yes or no. One particular patient replied, "No, I just lay there."

"You Should Have Twice as Much Fun"

I saw a new patient in consultation referred from a nurse practitioner. The history was nebulous when my nurse interviewed her and asked why she was there. I went in to see her and introduced myself. I asked what I could do for her. She said all she knew was that the nurse practitioner who referred her said she should be having twice as much fun. What in the world did that mean? We weren't sure what was going on.

I did a complete history and then an examination, and it then became obvious. She had two vaginas—a complete duplication of the mullerian system. I explained it to the couple, who said neither knew. There were two vaginas, two cervices, and two uteri. An ovary and tube were found by ultrasound lateral to each uterus.

She did need two pap smears.